Overview Map Key

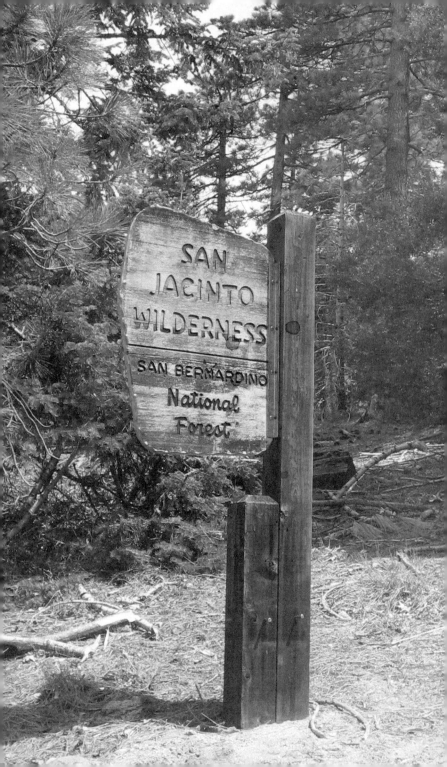

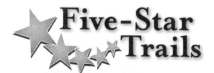

Five-Star Trails

Palm Springs

31 Spectacular Hikes in the Southern California Desert Resort Area

Laura Randall

MENASHA RIDGE PRESS
menasharidge.com

Five-Star Trails: Palm Springs

Copyright © 2016 by Laura Randall
All rights reserved
Published by Menasha Ridge Press
Printed in the United States of America
Distributed by Publishers Group West
First edition, first printing

Project editor: Ritchey Halphen
Cover design: Scott McGrew
Text design: Annie Long
Cover photos: Laura Randall; interior photos: as noted on page
Cartography and elevation profiles: Scott McGrew and Laura Randall
Copyeditor: Emily C. Beaumont
Proofreaders: Susan Elliott Brown (text), Dan Downing (maps and photo research)
Indexer: Sylvia Coates

Frontispiece: The San Jacinto Wilderness near Palm Springs offers nearly 50 miles of hiking trails that traverse a wide range of scenery, from desert canyons to pine-studded mountains. (Photo: Laura Randall)

Library of Congress Cataloging-in-Publication Data

Names: Randall, Laura, 1967– author.
Title: Five-star trails, Palm Springs / Laura Randall.
Description: First Edition. | Birmingham, Alabama : Menasha Ridge Press, [2016]
 "Distributed by Publishers Group West"—T.p. verso. | Includes index.
Identifiers: LCCN 2015043800 | ISBN 978-163404-038-9
 ISBN 978-163404-039-6 (e-book)
Subjects: LCSH: Hiking—California—Palm Springs Area—Guidebooks. | Trails—California—Palm Springs Area—Guidebooks. | Palm Springs Area (Calif.)—Guidebooks.
Classification: LCC GV199.42.C22 P347 2016 | DDC 796.510979497—dc23
LC record available at **lccn.loc.gov/2015043800**

MENASHA RIDGE PRESS
An imprint of AdventureKEEN
2204 1st Ave. S., Suite 102, Birmingham, AL 35233
800-443-7227, fax 205-326-1012

Visit **menasharidge.com** for a complete listing of our books and for ordering information. Contact us at our website, at **facebook.com/menasharidge**, or at **twitter.com/menasharidge** with questions or comments. To find out more about who we are and what we're doing, visit our blogs, **blog.menasharidge.com** and **blog.wildernesspress.com**.

Disclaimer This book is meant only as a guide to select trails in and around Palm Springs, California, and does not guarantee your safety in any way—you hike at your own risk. Do not attempt to explore terrain that may be beyond your abilities (such as areas with steep inclines or drop-offs). Please read carefully the introduction to this book, as well as safety information from other sources. Familiarize yourself with current weather reports and maps of the area you plan to visit (in addition to the maps provided in this guidebook). Be cognizant of park regulations, and always follow them. Also, note that land and road conditions, phone numbers and websites, and other information are subject to change.

Table of Contents

Coachella Valley Preserve 113

Santa Rosa and San Jacinto Mountains 129

Dedication

For John

Acknowledgments

THANKS TO THE FOLLOWING FOLKS for helping to make this book a reality: Jim Foote and the staff at the Palm Springs–South Coast field office of the Bureau of Land Management, the rangers at the Idyllwild Ranger Station, and Sarah Hahne and the Palm Springs Bureau of Tourism. Thanks also to all the folks at Menasha Ridge Press for their help, patience, and encouragement.

Thanks also to Julie Makinen, Mark Magers, and Linda Yoshino for hitting the trails with me, and to the Coachella Valley and Desert Trails Hiking Clubs for organizing regular hikes in the Palm Springs area and welcoming anyone who wants to join them. Most of all, thanks to John Kimble, who introduced me to Palm Springs two decades ago on a whirlwind weekend punctuated by thrift-store visits, sublime Mexican food, fresh air, and one unforgettable visit to the Salton Sea. Multiple trips later, my awe and appreciation of the Southern California desert haven't diminished one bit.

—*Laura Randall*

Preface

PALM SPRINGS OFTEN BRINGS TO MIND images of palm-lined golf courses and swimming pools surrounded by lounge chairs, not rugged hiking trails for people of all ages and fitness levels. Yet the striking mountain ranges that frame this desert resort are full of winding trails that lead to natural palm groves, year-round waterfalls and streams, and cactus-spiked desert terrain. It may be near two other great natural spaces—Joshua Tree National Park and Anza-Borrego Desert State Park—but the Palm Springs area is a hiking destination in its own right. The **Indian Canyons,** where the Agua Caliente tribe of Cahuilla Indians once spent their summers, have dozens of trails, from easy half-mile jaunts to arduous treks that link to the 2,650-mile Pacific Crest Trail and Idyllwild on the other side of the San Jacinto Mountains. Four of the canyons—**Palm, Andreas, Murray,** and **Fern**—are clustered together at the south end of town; another, **Tahquitz,** sits just off Palm Canyon Drive, Palm Springs' main drag.

To the north, the preserves of the **Coachella Valley** and **Big Morongo Canyon** are lovingly cared-for oases of palm groves, canyon washes, and tidal marshes that stand as testaments to the importance and dedication of volunteers. And in **Palm Springs** and neighboring towns like **Palm Desert** and **Rancho Mirage,** officials have worked with the Bureau of Land Management and others to improve and expand a network of trails while also keeping the area safe for the many forms of wildlife that inhabit it.

Desert trails come with their own unique sets of challenges. Hiking many of them during the summer months, when temperatures hit the triple digits, isn't a rational option for novice hikers. Parts of the Santa Rosa and San Jacinto Mountains are prime habitat for the endangered peninsular bighorn sheep, and many trails are closed to dogs year-round. Other areas are closed to all hikers during lambing season from January to June. I've noted this for individual

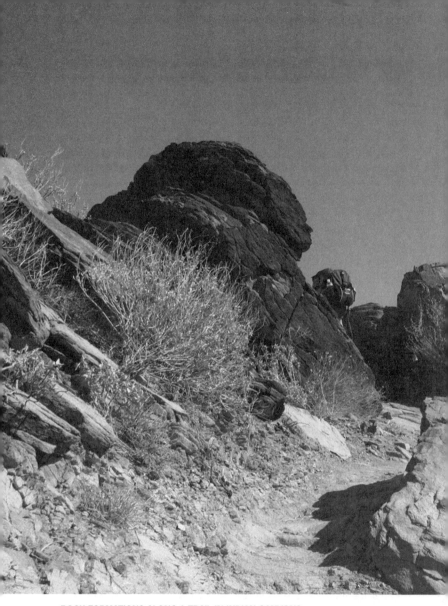

ROCK FORMATIONS ALONG A TRAIL IN INDIAN CANYONS   Photo: Laura Randall

trails, but it's always good to check with the Bureau of Land Management (**blm.gov**) or local recreation departments before hiking in or near a sensitive habitat.

None of the trails in Palm Springs and the other desert cities in this book allow overnight camping, but the nearby Santa Rosa and San Jacinto Mountains offer good camping options. **Idyllwild,** a small mountain town with four seasons and many charming inns and shops, is a scenic 40-mile drive away and may be used as a base for these hikes. Nearby, the densely forested mountains and cool, pine-scented air offer a striking balance to the rocky hillsides and sandy washes that dominate many of the Palm Springs trails.

This book offers 31 hikes within less than an hour's drive of Palm Springs. Some of them, like San Jacinto Peak (Hike 30) and the Lykken trails (Hikes 9 and 11), have been around for decades and have been described with adoration by everyone from John Muir to nature-loving bloggers. Other hikes, like Hopalong Cassidy (Hike 17) and the trails at Whitewater Preserve (Hike 15), are either newly developed or out of the way—they offer new and different experiences for even longtime hikers in the area. Whitewater Preserve, for instance, opened in 2008 and features a shady picnic area and pristine moderate trails that link up with the Pacific Crest Trail. As in Idyllwild, temperatures here are often 10–20 degrees cooler than they are in Palm Springs, making it a year-round hiking destination.

Whatever the reason you've chosen to visit or live in the Palm Springs area, hiking its trails will give you a real appreciation for the area's natural history and the way things were long before Frank Sinatra and the Rat Pack showed up. From the herds of bighorn sheep that still roam the hillsides to the hidden palm oases that helped the Agua Caliente Indians survive the searing summer heat centuries ago, there's much more going on around this stark desert landscape than one could ever initially imagine.

Recommended Hikes

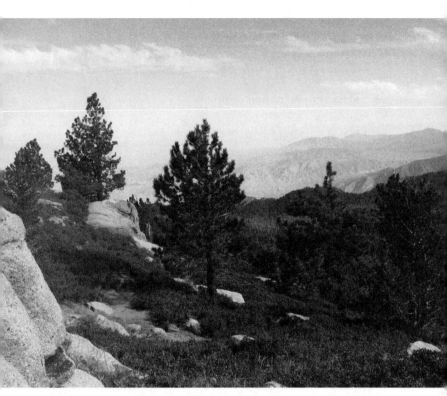

PINE FOREST AND MOUNTAIN VIEWS ALONG THE TRAIL TO SAN JACINTO PEAK
(See Hike 30, page 159.)   Photo: Laura Randall

Best for Children

Best for Dogs

Steep Hikes

Flat Hikes

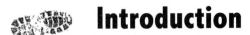 # Introduction

How to Use This Guidebook

The following section walks you through this book's organization, making it easy and convenient to plan great hikes.

The Overview Map, Overview Map Key, and Legend

The overview map on the inside front cover shows the primary trailheads for all 31 hikes. The numbers on the overview map pair with the map key on the facing page. A legend explaining the map symbols used throughout the book appears on the inside back cover.

Trail Maps

In addition to the overview map on the inside cover, a detailed map of each hike's route appears with its profile. On each of these maps, symbols indicate the trailhead, the complete route, significant features, facilities, and topographic landmarks such as creeks, overlooks, and peaks.

To produce the highly accurate maps in this book, I used a handheld GPS unit to gather data while hiking each route, then sent that data to Menasha Ridge Press's expert cartographers. Be aware, though, that your GPS device is no substitute for sound, sensible navigation that takes into account the conditions that you observe while hiking.

Further, despite the high quality of the maps in this guidebook, the publisher and I strongly recommend that you always carry an additional map, such as the ones noted in each profile opener's "Maps" entry.

Elevation Profile

Each hike includes this graphical element in addition to a trail map. Entries for fairly flat routes, such as a lake loop, do *not* display an elevation profile. Each entry's key information also lists the elevation at the trailhead.

The elevation diagram represents the rises and falls of the trail as viewed from the side, over the complete distance (in miles) of that trail. On the diagram's vertical axis, or height scale, the number of feet indicated between each tick mark lets you visualize the climb. To avoid making flat hikes look steep and steep hikes appear flat, varying height scales provide an accurate image of each hike's climbing challenge.

The Hike Profile

Each profile opens with the hike's star ratings, GPS trailhead coordinates, and other key at-a-glance information—from the trail's distance and configuration to contacts for local information. Each profile also includes a map (see "Trail Maps," page 1). The main text for each profile includes four sections: Overview, Route Details, Nearby Attractions (where applicable), and Directions (for driving to the trailhead area).

STAR RATINGS

The hikes in *Five-Star Trails: Palm Springs* were carefully chosen to give the hiker an overall five-star experience and represent the diversity of trails found in the region. Each hike was assigned a one- to five-star rating in each of the following categories: scenery, trail condition, suitability for children, level of difficulty, and degree of solitude. While one hike may merit five stars for its stunning scenery, that same trail may rank as a two-star trail for children. Similarly, another hike might receive two stars for difficulty but earn five stars for solitude. It's rare that any trail receives five stars in all five categories; nevertheless, each trail offers excellence in at least one category, if not others.

Here's how the star ratings for each of the five categories break down:

FOR SCENERY:

★ ★ ★ ★ ★   Unique, picturesque panoramas

★ ★ ★ ★   Diverse vistas

★ ★ ★   Pleasant views

★ ★   Unchanging landscape

★   Not selected for scenery

FOR TRAIL CONDITION:

★ ★ ★ ★ ★   Consistently well maintained

★ ★ ★ ★   Stable, with no surprises

★ ★ ★   Average terrain to negotiate

★ ★   Inconsistent, with good and poor areas

★   Rocky, overgrown, or often muddy

FOR CHILDREN:

★ ★ ★ ★ ★   Babes in strollers are welcome

★ ★ ★ ★   Fun for anyone past the toddler stage

★ ★ ★   Good for young hikers with proven stamina

★ ★   Not enjoyable for children

★   Not recommended for children

FOR DIFFICULTY:

★ ★ ★ ★ ★   Grueling

★ ★ ★ ★   Strenuous

★ ★ ★   Moderate: won't beat you up—but you'll know you've been hiking

★ ★   Easy with patches of moderate

★   Good for a relaxing stroll

FOR SOLITUDE:

★ ★ ★ ★ ★   Positively tranquil

★ ★ ★ ★   Spurts of isolation

★ ★ ★   Moderately secluded

★ ★   Crowded on weekends and holidays

★   Steady stream of individuals and/or groups

GPS TRAILHEAD COORDINATES

As noted in "Trail Maps," page 1, I used a handheld GPS unit to obtain geographic data and sent the information to the publisher's cartographers. In the opener for each hike profile, the coordinates—the intersection of the latitude (north) and longitude (west)—will orient you from the trailhead. In some cases, you can drive within viewing distance of a trailhead. Other hiking routes require a short walk to the trailhead from a parking area.

This guidebook expresses GPS coordinates in degree–decimal minute format. The latitude–longitude grid system is likely quite familiar to you, but here's a refresher, pertinent to visualizing the coordinates:

Imaginary lines of latitude—called *parallels* and located approximately 69 miles apart from each other—run horizontally around the globe. The equator is established to be 0°, and each parallel is indicated by degrees from the equator: up to 90°N at the North Pole and down to 90°S at the South Pole.

Imaginary lines of longitude—called *meridians*—run perpendicular to latitude lines. Longitude lines are likewise indicated by degrees. Starting from 0° at the Prime Meridian in Greenwich, England, they continue to the east and west until they meet 180° later at the International Date Line in the Pacific Ocean. At the equator, longitude lines also are approximately 69 miles apart, but that distance narrows as the meridians converge toward the North and South Poles.

To convert GPS coordinates given in degrees, minutes, and seconds to the format shown above in degrees–decimal minutes, the seconds are divided by 60. For more on GPS technology, visit **usgs.gov.**

DISTANCE AND CONFIGURATION

Distance notes the length of the hike round-trip, from start to finish. If the hike description includes options to shorten or extend the hike, those round-trip distances are also included here. *Configuration* defines the type of route—for example, an out-and-back (which takes you in and out the same way), a point-to-point (or one-way route), a figure-eight, or a balloon.

HIKING TIME

Two miles per hour is a general rule of thumb for the hiking times noted in this guidebook. That pace typically allows time for taking photos, for dawdling and admiring views, and for alternating stretches of hills and descents. When deciding whether or not to follow a particular trail in this guidebook, consider the weather, plus your own pace, general physical condition, and energy level on a given day.

HIGHLIGHTS
Lists features that draw hikers to the trail: mountain or forest views, water features, historic sites, and the like.

ELEVATION GAIN
In each trail's opener, you will see the elevation gain (in feet) at the trailhead. Each hike profile also includes an elevation diagram (see page 1).

ACCESS
Trail-access hours are listed here, along with any fees or permits required to hike the trail. Trails without fees or hours listed have free 24/7 access.

MAPS
Resources for maps, in addition to those in this guidebook, are listed here. As noted earlier, we recommend that you carry more than one map—and that you consult those maps before heading out on the trail in order to resolve any confusion or discrepancy.

FACILITIES
Includes visitor centers, restrooms, water, picnic tables, and other basics at or near the trailhead.

WHEELCHAIR ACCESS
Notes paved sections or other areas where one can safely use a wheelchair.

COMMENTS
Here you'll find assorted nuggets of information, such as whether or not dogs are allowed on the trails.

CONTACTS
Listed here are phone numbers and website addresses for checking trail conditions and gleaning other day-to-day information.

Overview, Route Details, Nearby Attractions, and Directions

These four elements compose the heart of the hike. "Overview" gives you a quick summary of what to expect on that trail; "Route Details" guides you on the hike, from start to finish; and "Nearby Attractions" suggests appealing adjacent sites, such as restaurants, museums, and other trails (note that not every hike profile has these). "Directions" will get you to the trailhead from a well-known road or highway.

Weather

Sunshine, low humidity, and high temperatures are the hallmarks of Palm Springs weather. The average annual rainfall is less than 10 inches. Winter days are mild, though strong winds can sometimes make hiking challenging, especially to the area west and north of town around San Gorgonio Pass. Temperatures start climbing in April and May and routinely exceed 100°F during the summer months. The risk of wildfires is also extremely high. Hiking during those times is not recommended. Layered clothing is a good idea when hiking between September and May. Temperatures can fluctuate on the trails as you weave in and out of canyons and the mountains cast late-afternoon shadows across the terrain.

Air quality tends to be good overall because the mountains surrounding the area serve as a barrier to the smog that plagues the Los Angeles basin.

Average Temperature by Month: Palm Springs					
	JAN	**FEB**	**MAR**	**APR**	**MAY**	**JUN**
High	70°F	75°F	80°F	88°F	95°F	104°F
Low	44°F	47°F	51°F	56°F	63°F	70°F
	JUL	**AUG**	**SEP**	**OCT**	**NOV**	**DEC**
High	108°F	107°F	101°F	91°F	78°F	70°F
Low	76°F	76°F	71°F	61°F	50°F	43°F

The chart on the previous page lists average monthly temperatures in Palm Springs. As noted earlier, temperatures in Idyllwild and around the San Jacinto Mountains can vary considerably and dip well below those reflected in the chart.

In general, the desert recreational season begins in October, when temperatures begin heading back down to the double digits and the lows hover at or above 60. By mid-November–February, tent camping becomes more challenging as temperatures begin dipping into the low 40s at night.

Water

A hiker walking steadily in 90-degree heat needs about 10 quarts of fluid per day. That's 2.5 gallons—12 large water bottles or 16 small ones. A good rule of thumb is to hydrate before your hike, carry (and drink) 6 ounces of water for every mile you plan to hike, and hydrate again after the hike.

For most people, the pleasures of hiking make carrying water a relatively minor burden, so pack more water than you anticipate needing, even for short hikes. If you don't like drinking tepid water on a hot day, freeze a couple of bottles overnight. It's also a good idea to carry a bottle of sports drink such as Gatorade; the electrolytes replace essential salts that you sweat out.

If you find yourself tempted to drink "found water," proceed with extreme caution. Many ponds and lakes you'll encounter are fairly stagnant, and the water tastes terrible. Drinking such water presents inherent risks for thirsty trekkers. Giardia parasites contaminate many water sources and cause the absolutely awful intestinal ailment giardiasis, which can last for weeks after onset. For more information, visit the Centers for Disease Control and Prevention website: **cdc.gov/parasites/giardia.**

In any case, effective treatment is essential before you use any water source found along the trail. Boiling water for 2–3 minutes is always a safe measure for camping, but day hikers can consider iodine tablets, approved chemical mixes, filtration units rated for giardia, and ultraviolet filtration. Some of these methods (for example, filtration with an added carbon filter) remove bad tastes typical in stagnant water, while others add their own taste. As a precaution, carry a means of water purification in case you've underestimated your consumption needs.

Clothing

Weather, unexpected trail conditions, fatigue, extended hiking duration, and wrong turns can individually or collectively turn a great outing into a very uncomfortable one at best—and a life-threatening one at worst. Thus, proper attire plays a key role in staying comfortable and, sometimes, in staying alive. Some helpful guidelines:

★ Choose silk, wool, or synthetics for maximum comfort in all of your hiking attire—from hats to socks and in between. Cotton is fine if the weather remains dry and stable, not so much if that material gets wet.

★ Always wear a hat, or at least tuck one into your day pack or hitch it to your belt. Hats offer all-weather sun and wind protection as well as warmth if it turns cold.

★ Be ready to layer up or down as the day progresses and the mercury rises or falls. Today's outdoor wear makes layering easy, with such designs as jackets that convert to vests and zip-off or button-up legs.

★ Wear hiking boots paired with good socks to avoid blisters. Flip-flopping along a paved urban greenway is one thing, but you should never hike a trail in open sandals or casual sneakers. Your bones and arches need support, and your skin needs protection from cacti along the trail. Plus, rattlesnakes, while rarely encountered, can't bite through hiking boots.

Essential Gear

Today you can buy outdoor vests that have up to 20 pockets shaped and sized to carry everything from toothpicks to binoculars. Or, if you don't aspire to feel like a burro, you can neatly stow all of these items in your day pack or backpack. The following list showcases never-hike-without-them items—in alphabetical order, as all are important:

★ *Extra clothes:* raingear (for the occasional rainy day), a change of socks, and depending on the season, a warm hat and gloves.

★ *Extra food:* trail mix, granola bars, or other high-energy snacks.

★ *Flashlight or headlamp* with extra bulb and batteries, for getting back to the trailhead if you take longer than expected.

★ *Insect repellent* to ward off ticks and other biting bugs.

★ *Maps and a high-quality compass.* Even if you know the terrain from previous hikes, don't leave home without these tools. And, as previously noted, bring maps in addition to those in this guidebook, and consult your maps prior to the hike. If you're GPS-savvy, bring that device, too, but don't rely on it as your sole navigational tool—battery life is limited, after all—and be sure to check its accuracy against that of your maps and compass.

★ *Pocketknife and/or multitool.*

★ *Sun protection:* sunglasses with UV tinting, a sunhat with a wide brim, and sunscreen.

★ *Toilet paper* and a zip-top plastic bag to pack it out in.

★ *Water.* Again, bring more than you think you'll drink. Depending on your destination, you may want to bring a container and iodine or a filter for purifying water in case you run out.

★ *Whistle.* It could become your best friend in an emergency.

★ *Windproof matches and/or a lighter,* for real emergencies— please don't start a forest fire.

First-Aid Kit

In addition to the preceding items, those that follow may seem daunting to carry along for a day hike. But any paramedic will tell you that the products listed here—again, in alphabetical order, because all are important—are just the basics. The reality of hiking is that you can be out for a week of backpacking and acquire only a mosquito bite. Or you can hike for an hour, slip, and suffer a cut or broken bone. Fortunately, the items listed pack into a very small space. You may also purchase convenient prepackaged kits at your pharmacy or online.

★ Adhesive bandages

★ Antibiotic ointment (such as Neosporin)

★ Aspirin, acetaminophen (Tylenol), or ibuprofen (Advil)

★ Athletic tape

★ Blister kit (moleskin or an adhesive variety such as Spenco 2nd Skin)

★ Butterfly-closure bandages

★ Diphenhydramine (Benadryl), in case of allergic reactions

★ Elastic bandages (such as Ace) or joint wraps (such as Spenco)

★ Epinephrine in a prefilled syringe (EpiPen), typically by prescription only, for people known to have severe allergic reactions to hiking mishaps such as bee stings

★ Gauze (one roll and a half-dozen 4-by-4-inch pads)

★ Hydrogen peroxide or iodine

Note: Consider your intended terrain and the number of hikers in your party before you exclude any article listed above. A short stroll may not inspire you to carry a complete kit, but anything beyond that warrants precaution. When hiking alone, you should always be prepared for a medical need. And if you're a twosome or with a group, one or more people in your party should be equipped with first-aid material.

Hiking with Children

The Southern California desert, with its cacti, rough terrain, and near-constant heat, makes many of the hikes in this book unsuitable for children. Fit kids age 10 or older may be able to handle flat, short trails, but the often-remote locations, coupled with the lack of shade and unforgiving climate, make hiking with toddlers and infants inappropriate. Use common sense to judge a child's capacity to hike a particular trail. Four hikes suitable for children are listed on page xiii.

General Safety

The desert can be a barren, intimidating place, but to those who take the time to prepare and explore this vast wilderness, the area reveals its natural treasure. Potential dangerous situations can occur, but preparation and sound judgment usually result in safe forays, even in remote areas. Here are a few tips to make your trip safer and easier:

★ *Always let someone know where you'll be hiking and how long you expect to be gone.* It's a good idea to give that person a copy of your route, particularly if you're headed into any isolated area. Let him or her know when you return.

★ *Always sign in and out of any trail registers provided.* Don't hesitate to comment on the trail condition if space is provided; that's your opportunity to alert others to any problems you encounter.

★ *Don't count on a mobile phone for your safety.* Reception may be spotty or nonexistent on the trail, even on an urban walk—especially one embraced by towering trees.

★ *Always carry food and water, even for a short hike.* And bring more water than you think you'll need. (We can't emphasize this enough!)

★ *Ask questions.* Public-land employees are on hand to help. It's a lot easier to solicit advice before a problem occurs, and it will help you avoid a mishap away from civilization when it's too late to amend an error.

★ *Stay on designated trails.* Even on the most clearly marked trails, you usually reach a point where you have to stop and consider in which direction to head. If you become disoriented, don't panic. As soon as you think you may be off-track, stop, assess your current direction, and then retrace your steps to the point where you went astray. Using a map, a compass, and this book, and keeping in mind what you've passed thus far, reorient yourself, and trust your judgment on which way to continue. If you become absolutely unsure of how to continue, return to your vehicle the way you came in. Should you become completely lost and have no idea how to find the trailhead, remaining in place along the trail and waiting for help is most often the best option for adults and always the best option for children.

★ *Always carry a whistle,* another precaution that we can't overemphasize. It may become a lifesaver if you get lost or hurt.

★ *Be especially careful when crossing streams.* Whether you're ford-ing the stream or crossing on a log, make every step count. If you have any doubt about maintaining your balance on a log, ford the stream instead: use a trekking pole or stout stick for balance and *face upstream as you cross.* If a stream seems too deep to ford, turn back. Whatever is on the other side isn't worth risking your life for.

★ *Be careful at overlooks.* While these areas may provide spectacular views, they are potentially hazardous. Stay back from the edge of outcrops, and make absolutely sure of your footing—a misstep can mean a nasty and possibly fatal fall.

★ *Standing dead trees and storm-damaged living trees pose a signifi-cant hazard to hikers.* These trees may have loose or broken limbs that could fall at any time. While walking beneath trees, and when choosing a spot to rest or enjoy your snack, *look up.*

★ *Know the symptoms of subnormal body temperature, or hypothermia.* Shivering and forgetfulness are the two most common indicators of this stealthy killer. Hypothermia can occur at any elevation, even in the sum-mer, especially if you're wearing lightweight cotton clothing. If symptoms develop, get to shelter, hot liquids, and dry clothes as soon as possible.

★ *Likewise, know the symptoms of heat exhaustion, or hyperthermia.* Here's how to recognize and handle three types of heat emergencies:

 ★ **Heat cramps** are painful cramps in the leg and abdomen, accom-panied by heavy sweating and feeling faint. Caused by excessive salt loss, heat cramps must be handled by getting to a cool place and sip-ping water or an electrolyte solution (such as Gatorade).

 ★ Dizziness, headache, irregular pulse, disorientation, and nausea are all symptoms of **heat exhaustion,** which occurs as blood vessels dilate and attempt to move heat from the inner body to the skin. Find a cool place, drink cool water, and get a friend to fan you, which can help cool you off more quickly.

 ★ Dilated pupils; dry, hot, flushed skin; a rapid pulse; high fever; and abnormal breathing are all symptoms of **heatstroke,** a life-threatening condition that can cause convulsions, unconsciousness, or even death. If you should be sweating and you're not, that's the signature warning sign. If you or a hiking partner is experiencing heatstroke, do whatever you can to cool down and find help.

★ *Most importantly, take along your brain.* A cool, calculating mind is the single most important asset on the trail. Think before you act.

Watch your step. Plan ahead. Avoiding accidents before they happen is the best way to ensure a rewarding and relaxing hike.

Watchwords for Flora and Fauna

TICKS These arachnids are commonly found in brushy and wooded areas. Therefore, you are less likely to encounter them in desert areas than in other regions. Ticks need a host to feed on in order to reproduce. The ones that alight on you while you hike will be very small, sometimes so tiny that you won't be able to spot them. Primarily of two varieties, deer ticks and dog ticks, both need a few hours of actual attachment before they can transmit any disease they may harbor. Ticks may settle in shoes, socks, or hats, and they may take several hours to actually latch on. The best strategy is to visually check every half-hour or so while hiking, do a thorough check before you get in the car, and then, when you take a posthike shower, do an even more thorough check of your entire body. Remove ticks that are already embedded using tweezers made for this purpose. Treat the bite with disinfectant solution.

SNAKES Several types of rattlesnakes inhabit the Palm Springs region. I've never encountered one while hiking, but you should always be on the lookout for them. If you see one, give it plenty of

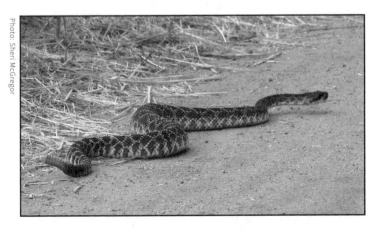

Photo: Sheri McGregor

room and leave it alone. When snakes have the opportunity, they slither out of sight before you are upon them. Because snakes sense vibrations, pounding a hiking stick along the ground as you walk gives them fair warning of your presence and allows them to escape. Don't step or put your hands where you can't see, and avoid wandering around in the dark. Step *onto* logs and rocks, never *over* them, and be especially careful when climbing rocks. Avoid walking through dense brush whenever possible. As with any wild animal, snakes are drawn to available water, so you may be more likely to encounter them near streams.

MOUNTAIN LIONS Also known as pumas or cougars, these big cats reside in the San Jacinto and Santa Rosa Mountains, and they have occasionally been spotted in the brushy foothills and riparian areas adjacent to them. Encounters are rare, but whenever you venture into an animal's habitat, the possibility exists. A few guidelines:

★ *Keep children close to you, or hold your child.* Observed in captivity, mountain lions seem especially drawn to small children.

★ *Do not approach a mountain lion.* Instead, give it room to get away.

★ *Try to make yourself look larger* by raising your arms and opening your jacket if you're wearing one.

★ *Don't crouch or kneel.* These movements could make you look smaller and more like the lion's prey.

★ *Try to convince the lion that you're dangerous—not its prey.* With as little movement as possible, gather nearby stones or branches and toss them at the animal. Slowly wave your arms above your head and speak in a firm voice.

★ *If all fails and you get attacked, fight back.* Hikers have successfully fought off an attacking lion with rocks and sticks. Try to remain facing the animal, and fend off attempts to bite at your head or neck— a lion's typical aim.

POISON OAK Although uncommon, poison oak does exist in the desert. Where water is present, you may find poison oak—recognized by its three-leaflet configuration *(see photo)*—on either a vine or shrub.

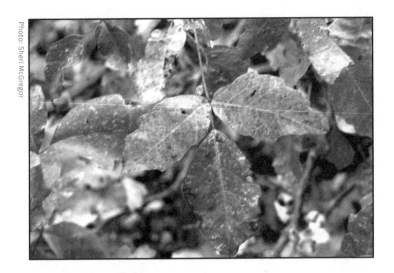

Photo: Sheri McGregor

Urushiol, the oil in the sap of this plant, is responsible for the rash. Usually within 12–14 hours of exposure (but sometimes much later), raised lines and/or blisters will appear, accompanied by a terrible itch. Try to refrain from scratching, though, because bacteria under your fingernails can cause an infection. Wash and dry the rash thoroughly, applying calamine lotion or another product to help dry the rash. If itching or blistering is severe, seek medical attention. To keep from spreading the misery to someone else, wash not only any exposed parts of your body but also any oil-contaminated clothes, hiking gear, and pets. Long pants and a long-sleeved shirt may offer the best protection.

PENINSULAR BIGHORN SHEEP These sheep inhabit dry, rocky, low-elevation desert slopes, canyons, and washes from the San Jacinto and Santa Rosa mountains near Palm Springs, California, south into Baja California, Mexico. They have been listed under the California State Endangered Species Act (ESA) since 1971, but their population has seen a slow but steady rise in the last decade. Helicopter surveys conducted in 2004 indicated that approximately 700 Peninsular bighorns inhabited the United States. By 2015, the California Department of Fish and Wildlife estimated that the number had grown to

915, many of them dwelling in the hills above La Quinta, Rancho Mirage, and Palm Desert. The Palm Springs–South Coast Field Office of the Bureau of Land Management restricts dogs and hiking during sensitive times of the year, such as summer and lambing season in areas frequented by bighorn sheep.

The lambing season for bighorn sheep occurs between January 1 and September 30; during this time, hikers are required to remain on the trails, and some trails, like Clara Burgess and Art Smith, prohibit dogs year-round for fear that they will drive the sheep from the area.

If you do spot a bighorn sheep in the area (but not on the trail), just continue walking at a steady pace along the trail. If the sheep is on or immediately adjacent to the trail (a rare thing), the Bureau of Land Management advises stopping and allowing the sheep to move off the trail of its own accord. Don't try to shoo or herd the sheep off the trail.

Tips for Enjoying Palm Springs and Idyllwild

Though most of these hikes are within easy reach of downtown Palm Springs and CA 111, it's easy to get lost or disoriented on the trails. Many of them quickly cut you off from civilization and disappear around mountain ridges and through thick desert vegetation. Know the trail and its surroundings before you go. Good maps are available at the visitor centers in Palm Springs and Palm Desert, as well as the visitor center for the Santa Rosa and San Jacinto Mountains National Monument on CA 74. The staff at these visitor centers will be happy to brief you on what to expect in terms of trail condition, history, and wildlife.

Also stop by the Idyllwild Ranger Station before setting off. The office has good trail maps, camping information, and knowledgeable staff. This is also the place to pick up wilderness and camping permits for trails like Devil's Slide and San Jacinto Peak, as well as the National Forest Adventure Pass (see "Backcountry Advice," opposite).

Here are a few more tips for enjoying your time in the mountains and desert:

★ *Take your time along the trails.* Pace yourself. The mountains and desert around Palm Springs are filled with wonders big and small. Don't rush past a jackrabbit or cluster of ocotillo trees to get to that final overlook. Stop and smell the wildflowers, if you're lucky enough to experience them after a rainy winter. Take time to revel in the cool shade of the towering palm groves you'll encounter on many of these trails.

★ *Get an early start on the longer hikes,* especially in winter, so you don't have to rush to make it back to the trailhead before dark. Late afternoon is a perfect time for shorter hikes, as the air cools in winter and early spring and the sun casts dramatic shadows over the stark brown mountainsides. That said, take close notice of the elevation maps that accompany each hike. If you see many large altitude changes, allow for extra time. Inevitably, you'll finish some of the hikes long before or after the times suggested in each profile. Nevertheless, leave yourself plenty of time for those moments when you simply feel like stopping and taking it all in.

★ *Don't wander too far off the main trail* unless you've done your homework. Many unmarked paths branch off from the main trails around Palm Springs: Some eventually hook back up with the trail system; others dead-end at streams or sheer rock walls. If you're ever unsure, stick to the main trail (usually the one with the most footprints), and don't be afraid to ask other hikers for directions.

★ *Hike during the week.* We can't always schedule our free time when we want, but try to hike the busier trails, such as those in the Indian Canyons and Idyllwild's Devil's Slide Trail, on a weekday (though always with a companion). If you're hiking on a busy weekend, go early in the morning to enhance your chances of seeing wildlife and increase your chances of solitude. Finally, use common sense if hiking the Palm Springs trails during the summer or early fall: Get as early a start as possible, bring plenty of water and sunscreen, and avoid triple-digit-temperature days altogether.

Backcountry Advice

A permit is not required to hike any trails within the Palm Springs area, and overnight camping isn't allowed on any of the trails in the desert cities. The San Jacinto and Santa Rosa Mountains offer many campsites near the trails; many require a **National Forest Adventure Pass,** which costs $5 per day or $30 per year. Adventure Passes are available at sporting-goods stores and local ranger stations; visit **tinyurl.com/usfsadventurepass** for general information or **tinyurl.com /adventurepassvendors** for a vendor list. An **Interagency Annual Pass** ($80 per year) or **Interagency Senior Pass** ($10 lifetime, ages 62 and older) may be used in lieu of an Adventure Pass at any fee-charging Forest Service, National Park Service, Bureau of Land Management, Bureau of Reclamation, or US Fish & Wildlife Service site. Other day hikes around Idyllwild require that you pick up a free wilderness permit from the nearest ranger office before setting out. This is high-fire-hazard country; open fires are not allowed anywhere in the wilderness. Check with the Forest Service at 909-382-2922 for other restrictions and updates.

Solid human waste must be buried in a hole at least 3 inches deep and at least 200 feet away from trails and water sources; a trowel is a basic piece of backpacking equipment.

Following the above guidelines will increase your chances for a pleasant, safe, and low-impact interaction between humans and nature. The suggestions are intended to enhance your experience.

Trail Etiquette

Always treat trails, wildlife, and fellow hikers with respect. Here are some reminders:

★ *Plan ahead in order to be self-sufficient at all times.* For example, carry necessary supplies for changes in weather or other conditions. A well-planned trip brings satisfaction to you and others.

★ *Hike on open trails only.*

★ *Check conditions before you head out* if you know that road or trail closures may be a possibility (use the websites or phone numbers listed in the "Contacts" section at the beginning of each hike profile). And don't try to circumvent such closures.

★ *Don't trespass on private land,* and obtain all permits and authorization as required. Leave gates as you found them or as directed by signage.

★ *Be courteous to other hikers,* bikers, equestrians, and others you encounter on the trails.

★ *Never spook wild animals or pets.* An unannounced approach, a sudden movement, or a loud noise startles most critters, and a surprised animal can be dangerous to you, to others, and to itself. Give animals plenty of space.

★ *Observe any* YIELD *signs you encounter.* Typically they advise hikers to yield to horses, and bikers to yield to both horses and hikers. Observing common courtesy on hills, hikers and bikers yield to any uphill traffic. When encountering mounted riders or horsepackers, hikers can courteously step off the trail, on the downhill side if possible. So that horses can see and hear you, calmly greet their riders before they reach you, and don't dart behind trees. Also resist the urge to pet horses unless you are invited to do so.

★ *Stay on the existing trail,* and don't blaze any new trails.

★ *Practice **Leave No Trace** principles.* Leave the trail in the same shape you found it in, if not better. Visit **lnt.org** for more information.

Indian Canyons

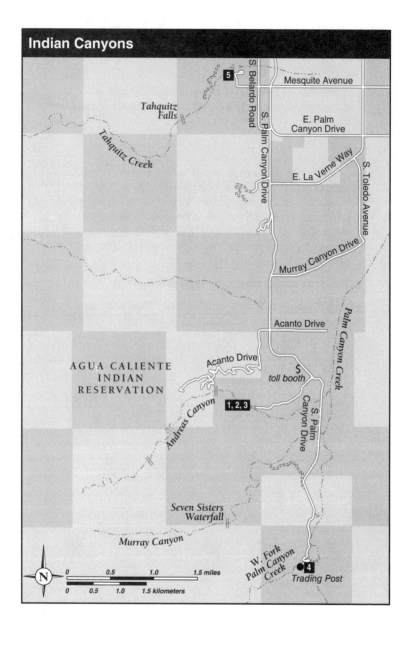

Tahquitz Falls

Tahquitz Creek

S. Belardo Road

5

Mesquite Avenue

S. Palm Canyon Drive

E. Palm Canyon Drive

E. La Verne Way

S. Toledo Avenue

Murray Canyon Drive

Acanto Drive

Palm Canyon Creek

AGUA CALIENTE
INDIAN
RESERVATION

Acanto Drive

$ toll booth

1, 2, 3

Andreas Canyon

S. Palm Canyon Drive

Seven Sisters
Waterfall

Murray Canyon

W. Fork
Palm Canyon
Creek

4

Trading Post

N

| 0 | 0.5 | 1.0 | 1.5 miles |

| 0 | 0.5 | 1.0 | 1.5 kilometers |

Indian Canyons

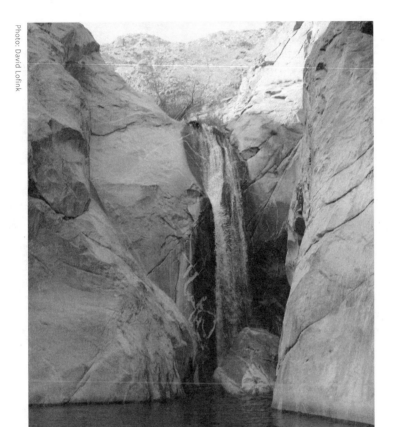

THIS 60-FOOT WATERFALL IS A HIGHLIGHT OF THE TAHQUITZ CANYON TRAIL.
(See Hike 5, page 41.)

Andreas Canyon Trail

SCENERY: ★ ★ ★ ★
TRAIL CONDITION: ★ ★ ★ ★
CHILDREN: ★ ★ ★ ★ ★
DIFFICULTY: ★
SOLITUDE: ★ ★

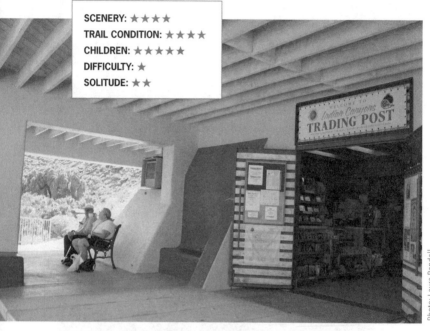

Photo: Laura Randall

THE INDIAN CANYONS TRADING POST IS A FAVORITE POSTHIKE STOP THAT SELLS COLD DRINKS, SNACKS, AND SOUVENIRS.

GPS TRAILHEAD COORDINATES: N33° 45.653' W116° 32.976'

DISTANCE & CONFIGURATION: 1- to 3-mile loop

HIKING TIME: 40 minutes–1 hour

HIGHLIGHTS: California fan palms, caves, unusual rock formations, year-round stream

ELEVATION GAIN: 285'

ACCESS: Open daily 8 a.m.–5 p.m. October–June, Friday–Sunday July–September. Admission: $9 per adult/$5 per child ages 6–12, payable at front gate.

MAPS: Detailed maps are posted at kiosks throughout the property and available at the entrance station and the Trading Post in Palm Canyon.

FACILITIES: Restrooms and picnic tables along the trail

WHEELCHAIR ACCESS: None

COMMENTS: No pets or bikes on trails. Gates close at 5 p.m., and no vehicles are allowed in after 4 p.m.

CONTACTS: 714-323-6018, **indian-canyons.com**

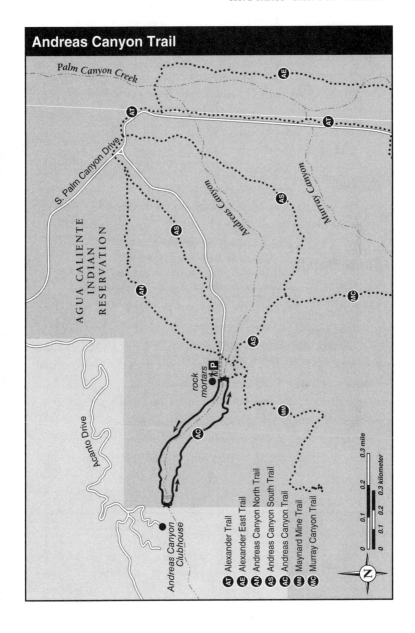

Andreas Canyon Trail

Palm Canyon Creek

S. Palm Canyon Drive

AGUA CALIENTE INDIAN RESERVATION

Andreas Canyon

Murray Canyon

rock mortars

Acanto Drive

Andreas Canyon Clubhouse

- AT Alexander Trail
- AE Alexander East Trail
- AN Andreas Canyon North Trail
- AS Andreas Canyon South Trail
- AC Andreas Canyon Trail
- MM Maynard Mine Trail
- MC Murray Canyon Trail

0   0.1   0.2   0.3 mile
0   0.1   0.2   0.3 kilometer

N

FIVE-STAR TRAILS

Overview

This short, scenic loop should be a part of any trip to the Indian Canyons. It's especially good for families, bird-watchers, and anyone who wants to experience the serenity of the canyons in a short period of time. The well-marked path leads past sheer rock walls and a year-round stream shaded by California fan palms to a seasonal waterfall and 1925 clubhouse once used by local hunters, then gives way to wide-open desert landscape. Though the best scenery can be found along the main 1-mile loop, the hike can be extended by 2 miles by picking up the easy horse trail on the north side of the road just before the parking lot entrance.

Route Details

The Indian Canyons, just south of downtown Palm Springs, are desert oases and the ancestral home of the Agua Caliente band of Cahuilla Indians. The area boasts year-round waterfalls, rocky canyon streams, and some of the largest collections of California fan palm oases in the world. More than a dozen trails of all levels snake through the canyons and connect to trails in Palm Springs and as far away as Idyllwild. Remnants of ancient life, such as irrigation ditches, stone shelters, and rock art, can be found along many of the trails. The entrance fees prohibit the area from being a regular hiking venue for area residents, but it's worth a visit at least once for anyone who

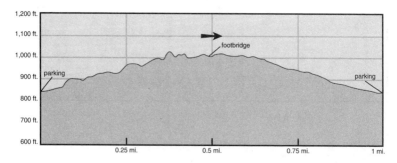

wants to combine a hike with pristine desert landscapes and insights into an ancient culture.

Look for the Andreas Canyon trailhead at the north end of the parking lot, just past a cluster of large rock formations. There is a sign on the right just before the trailhead that marks an Indian grinding mortar. The Cahuilla Indians used the bedrock mortars in front of you to grind mesquite beans, acorns, and wild oats.

Follow the packed sand-and-rock trail down a gradual hill past more rock formations. The stream, shaded by oaks, palms, and other trees, is to your left. This is a great place for kids to splash around and boulder-hop, especially in summer and fall, when water levels are low. In the fall, the leaves on some of the trees turn bright yellow and orange, making a nice contrast to the lush green palm trees.

The trail continues flat between the stream and towering rock formations. At 0.25 mile, pass a signpost for Andreas Canyon and take the path under a natural arch made of desert scrub brush. Continue straight along the flat trail, with the stream to your left. Soon the trail makes a brief ascent, then descends some natural rock steps and comes within touching distance of more California fan palms before hugging a sheer rock wall. Look for a small cave on the right— the Cahuilla Indians once used this and other small caves in the area for shelter. At almost 0.5 mile, the stream gives way to a pretty waterfall flanked by large boulders, another great place to stop and rest or have a picnic. I hiked this trail in the fall, when water levels were low, but the boulders can be slippery in late spring or after it rains. Be sure to wear sturdy shoes, just in case.

To the west of the waterfall are two small stone buildings on a hill; a chain-link fence bars public access. One of the buildings is the Andreas Canyon Clubhouse, the headquarters for a hunting club formed in 1923 on land once owned by the Southern Pacific Railroad. According to a sign, club members camped in the nearby streambed, using caches made of rocks. From here the trail crosses a small wooden footbridge and loops back to the east; now the stream is to your left. Ascend a moderate flight of natural rock steps past distant views of rock formations and fields of creosote and desert sage. The trail levels for 0.25 mile before ending back at the parking lot.

The hike is best done in the winter or early spring because there is virtually no shade. Those who want to extend this hike can either hop on the Murray Canyon Trail south of the parking lot or pick up the Andreas Canyon Horse Trail to the east of the parking lot. The horse trail isn't as well marked as the main loop, but it's impossible to get lost, as the main road in and out of the canyon stays within sight the entire time.

Nearby Attractions

Downtown Palm Springs is only a few miles north, but the self-contained reservation seems worlds away from the bustle of Palm Canyon Drive. It's a good idea to bring a lunch and plenty of cold drinks to enjoy at the picnic tables near the trailheads before or after your hike. The **Trading Post,** near the Palm Canyon trailhead, sells cold drinks and snacks, as well as Southwest-themed trinkets. It's also the starting point for guided nature and history hikes on weekends October–June. Call ahead (714-323-6018) for times.

Directions

From southbound I-10, take Exit 111 and drive south 9.4 miles on CA 111 through downtown Palm Springs. Continue straight (south) on South Palm Canyon Drive for about 3 miles to the Indian Canyons toll gate, where you can pick up a map and pay the entrance fee. Turn right just after the entrance gate and go about a mile to the parking lot for Murray and Andreas Canyons.

Maynard Mine Trail

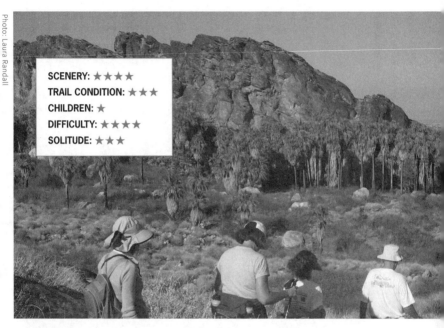

SCENERY: ★ ★ ★ ★
TRAIL CONDITION: ★ ★ ★
CHILDREN: ★
DIFFICULTY: ★ ★ ★ ★
SOLITUDE: ★ ★ ★

Photo: Laura Randall

HIKERS ENJOY EXPANSIVE VIEWS OF LARGE ROCK FORMATIONS AND PALM OASES ALONG THE TRAIL.

GPS TRAILHEAD COORDINATES: N33° 45.653' W116° 32.976'

DISTANCE & CONFIGURATION: 6-mile out-and-back

HIKING TIME: 4–5 hours

HIGHLIGHTS: Old tungsten mine, rock formations, desert vegetation, panoramic views

ELEVATION GAIN: 2,100'

ACCESS: Open daily 8 a.m.–5 p.m. October–June, Friday–Sunday July–September. Admission: $9 per adult/$5 per child ages 6–12, payable at front gate.

MAPS: Detailed maps are posted at kiosks throughout the property and available at the entrance station and the Trading Post in Palm Canyon.

FACILITIES: Restrooms and picnic tables along the trail

WHEELCHAIR ACCESS: None

COMMENTS: No pets or bikes on trails. Gates close at 5 p.m., and no vehicles are allowed in after 4 p.m.

CONTACTS: 714-323-6018, **indian-canyons.com**

Maynard Mine Trail

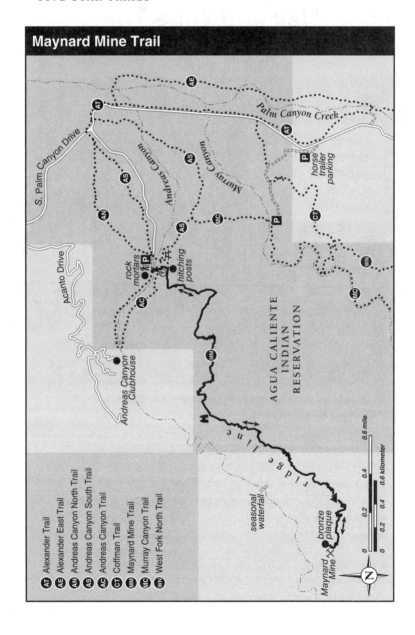

Palm Canyon Creek

horse trailer parking

S. Palm Canyon Drive

Andreas Canyon

Murray Canyon

Acanto Drive

rock mortars

hitching posts

AGUA CALIENTE INDIAN RESERVATION

Andreas Canyon Clubhouse

ridge line

seasonal waterfall

bronze plaque

Maynard Mine

AT	Alexander Trail
AE	Alexander East Trail
AN	Andreas Canyon North Trail
AS	Andreas Canyon South Trail
AC	Andreas Canyon Trail
CT	Coffman Trail
MM	Maynard Mine Trail
MC	Murray Canyon Trail
WN	West Fork North Trail

0   0.2   0.4   0.6 mile

0   0.2   0.4   0.6 kilometer

Overview

The Maynard Mine Trail is one of the more challenging trails within the Indian Canyons trail system. It once served as the access route for a tungsten mine that operated during World War II. It begins in Murray Canyon and climbs steadily to the top of a ridge separating Murray and Andreas canyons, then drops over to a razorback ridge that leads to the mine. Explore the mine and a few pieces of rusty equipment left behind, and enjoy the mountain and valley views before heading back. Sturdy hiking shoes and a hat and sunscreen are essential. Long pants are recommended because of the cacti and catclaw acacia plants that line the path.

Route Details

This out-and-back hike starts on the south side of the Andreas and Murray Canyons parking lot. Cross the small concrete bridge and look for a kiosk with a detailed map and a sign pointing you toward the Maynard Mine trailhead. Follow the path down a short hill to a row of horse-hitching posts, then make a sharp right and look for a large sign marked MAYNARD MINE. Follow the narrow loose-gravel path up the rock- and scrub-covered hillside. After 0.3 mile of uphill walking, you will start to see nice views of the mountains and Palm

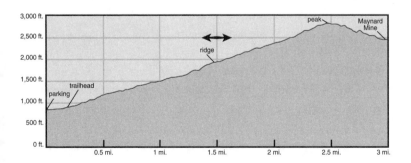

Springs. Be careful of the cholla cactus and catclaw acacia that can be found on either side of the path. Their short curved spines will cling to your clothes and can be very difficult to untangle.

At about 1.1 miles, the trail splits: Head straight to stay on the main path. (If you take the left path, you'll have to do some boulder scrambling over steep terrain to get back to the main path, and it will slow you down a bit.) At 1.5 miles, the trail reaches the mountain ridge and provides wide-open views of Andreas Canyon to the right. From here you can also see a long water pipeline snaking across the mountain ridge: This was once used by the Cahuilla Indians to deliver water into Andreas Canyon from mountain streams. To the far right are a few private homes perched on the mountain above the pipeline. Continue hiking south along a gradual incline up the ridge for another mile or so. If it's winter or early spring, look to the right across the canyon for a view of a waterfall. At 2.5 miles, you will come to a signpost for Maynard Mine. You are at the hike's peak elevation of 2,100 feet, and it's all downhill from here.

The trail now follows a razorback ridge for another 0.4 mile to a clearing marked by a pile of mine tailings and a bronze plaque dedicated to Jim Maynard, the miner who first had the guts to lug a wheelbarrow and shovel to the middle of a barren hillside and start digging. The actual mine is about 200 yards north. Over the hill to the west are a few pieces of equipment used by miners, including an air compressor. Many visitors like to rest and have lunch here because there are boulders for sitting and beautiful views of the mountains. To the southwest are Apache Peak, Antsell Rock, and Red Tahquitz Peak; the Pacific Crest Trail runs right below them.

In the fall, a small strip of deciduous trees that lines the canyon are ablaze with red and orange. From the clearing, a steep dirt and gravel path leads down to a pretty canyon stream framed by these trees, but it's not recommended that hikers go beyond the mine. From the mine, you'll have to retrace your steps back to the parking lot. The return is easier, more leisurely, and graced by expansive views of large rock formations, palm oases, and the city of Palm Springs.

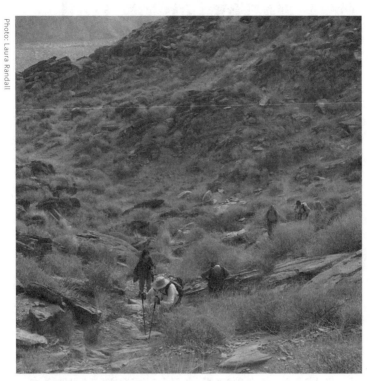

Photo: Laura Randall

CHOLLA CACTUS AND CATCLAW ACACIA GROW ON THE HILLS SURROUNDING THE TRAIL.

Nearby Attractions

See previous hike.

Directions

From southbound I-10, take Exit 111 and drive south 9.4 miles on CA 111 through downtown Palm Springs. Continue straight (south) on South Palm Canyon Drive for about 3 miles to the Indian Canyons toll gate, where you can pick up a map and pay the entrance fee. Turn right just after the entrance gate and go about a mile to the parking lot for Murray and Andreas Canyons.

Murray Canyon Trail

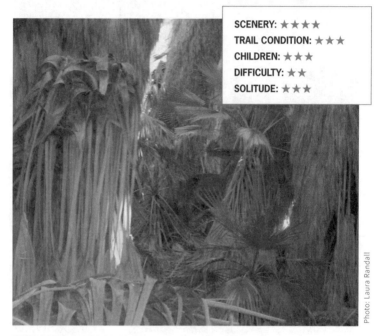

SCENERY: ★ ★ ★ ★
TRAIL CONDITION: ★ ★ ★
CHILDREN: ★ ★ ★
DIFFICULTY: ★ ★
SOLITUDE: ★ ★ ★

Photo: Laura Randall

THICK PALMS OFFER SOME SHADE ALONG THE MURRAY CANYON TRAIL.

GPS TRAILHEAD COORDINATES: N33° 45.653' W116° 32.976'

DISTANCE & CONFIGURATION: 4-mile out-and-back

HIKING TIME: 2 hours

HIGHLIGHTS: California fan palms, year-round stream with waterfalls, ancient rock formations

ELEVATION GAIN: 500'

ACCESS: Open daily 8 a.m.–5 p.m. October–June, Friday–Sunday July–September. Admission: $9 per adult/$5 per child ages 6–12, payable at front gate

MAPS: Detailed maps are posted at kiosks throughout the property and available at the entrance station and the Trading Post in Palm Canyon.

FACILITIES: Restrooms; picnic tables along the trail

WHEELCHAIR ACCESS: None

COMMENTS: No pets or bikes on trails. Gates close at 5 p.m., and no vehicles are allowed in after 4 p.m.

CONTACTS: 714-323-6018, **indian-canyons.com**

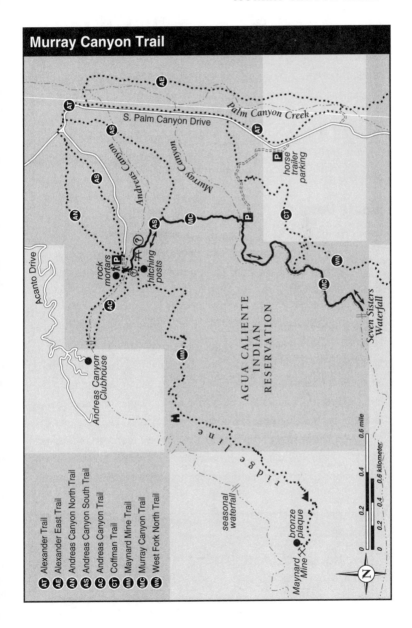

Murray Canyon Trail

AT Alexander Trail
AE Alexander East Trail
AN Andreas Canyon North Trail
AS Andreas Canyon South Trail
AC Andreas Canyon Trail
CT Coffman Trail
MM Maynard Mine Trail
MC Murray Canyon Trail
WN West Fork North Trail

Overview

Wear sturdy hiking shoes for this moderate but mostly flat hike in the Indian Canyons. After a brief dusty trek across sand and through desert scrub, the route weaves in and out of a stream lined with palms to reach a series of seasonal waterfalls known as Seven Sisters. Expect a moderate amount of rock scrambling and stream fording, especially in late winter and spring when water levels are higher. Keep an eye out for rattlesnakes during the warm summer months.

Route Details

From the parking lot, head south across the bridge to a kiosk with a map and trail information. Turn left at the kiosk and follow the unpaved fire road past a small palm grove with a few picnic tables to another kiosk with a sign for Murray Canyon/Seven Sisters. Take the sand-and-gravel trail straight beyond the kiosk as it begins a gradual descent into the canyon. After about 200 yards, the trail comes to a fork: Go right, following the signs for Murray Canyon; to the left is a short path that leads to the Andreas Canyon South Trail, a more strenuous hike that goes deep into the San Jacinto Mountains. The next quarter-mile is a flat walk past brown hillsides and desert vegetation, such as creosote bush, cottonwood trees, and lavender. At 0.6 mile, the scenery improves as the trail wanders among ragged boulders; you can see the palm oasis in the distance and large rock formations to the right. Palm Springs and the Little San Bernardino

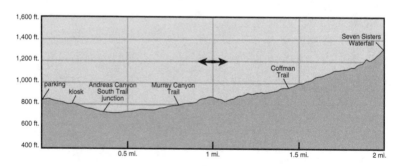

Mountains are north, in the distance. At 0.75 mile, the trail makes a brief descent into the palm oasis, and you'll reach the first of several stream crossings. This marks the beginning of Murray Canyon. Follow the signpost toward Seven Sisters to the right; the left fork (after the stream crossing) leads to the Coffman and West Fork Trails.

The remaining mile is the toughest part of the hike, as the path weaves in and out of the palm oasis and across big rocks. To the left are stunning copper-colored rock formations, piled high and at wacky angles—a great photo opportunity. From here the trail heads briefly into the shade of an arch of tall scrub brush, then continues east on a narrow, rocky course toward more palm trees.

At 1.2 miles, you'll come to another signpost for Seven Sisters. Beyond it, the trail continues its gradual ascent up a rocky hillside, with the palm oasis to the right, then heads down into the canyon. Now you are deep into the canyon, surrounded by California fan palms and natural pools—a world away from bustling Palm Springs. This trail gets a moderate amount of foot traffic, though, so don't be surprised to run into fellow hikers and even the occasional equestrian.

At 1.7 miles, the trail crosses the stream again and heads uphill in short, easy switchbacks before dipping back down into the canyon. After a brief, steep ascent of carved rock steps, the trail levels again. Be sure to stop here and look back for a fine bird's-eye view of Murray Canyon. You've reached Seven Sisters, a series of waterfalls fed by natural pools and shaded by California fan palms. Don't count on all the waterfalls to be flowing, especially in the dry fall months. The best time to see them is April or May, according to canyon rangers. The area is dotted with big, flat rocks, perfect for having a picnic lunch by the water. You can also hike down to the pools, or just make your way under the waterfalls for a unique view of the canyon.

From here make your way back to the main trail and retrace your route to the parking lot. There are also picnic tables near the parking area if you want to cap your hike with lunch or a snack.

Directions

From southbound I-10, take Exit 111 and drive south 9.4 miles on CA 111 through downtown Palm Springs. Continue straight (south) on South Palm Canyon Drive for about 3 miles to the Indian Canyons toll gate, where you can pick up a map and pay the entrance fee. Turn right just after the entrance gate and go about a mile to the parking lot for Murray and Andreas Canyons.

Palm Canyon Trail to the Stone Pools

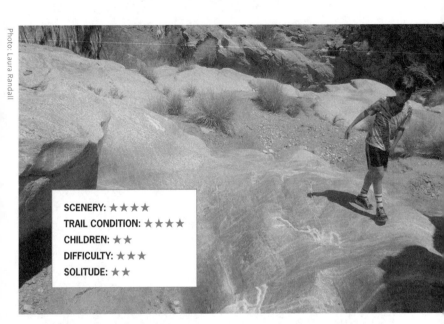

SCENERY: ★ ★ ★

TRAIL CONDITION: ★ ★ ★ ★

CHILDREN: ★ ★

DIFFICULTY: ★ ★ ★

SOLITUDE: ★ ★

THE STONE POOLS, A CLUSTER OF ROCK GORGES ALONG PALM CANYON TRAIL, OFFER SHADE AND SOMETIMES WATER FOR WEARY HIKERS.

GPS TRAILHEAD COORDINATES: N33° 44.279' W116° 32.348'

DISTANCE & CONFIGURATION: 5.8-mile out-and-back

HIKING TIME: 2.5–3 hours

HIGHLIGHTS: Palm oasis, San Jacinto Mountains backdrop

ELEVATION GAIN: 800'

ACCESS: Open daily 8 a.m.–5 p.m. October–June, Friday–Sunday July–September. Admission: $9 per adult/$5 per child ages 6–12, payable at front gate

MAPS: Detailed maps are posted at kiosks throughout the property and available at the entrance station and the Trading Post in Palm Canyon.

FACILITIES: Restrooms, snack bar, picnic tables

WHEELCHAIR ACCESS: None

COMMENTS: No pets or bikes on trails. Gates close at 5 p.m., and no vehicles are allowed to enter after 4 p.m. In summer (July–September), the Indian Canyons are open only Friday–Sunday.

CONTACTS: 714-323-6018, **indian-canyons.com**

Palm Canyon Trail to the Stone Pools

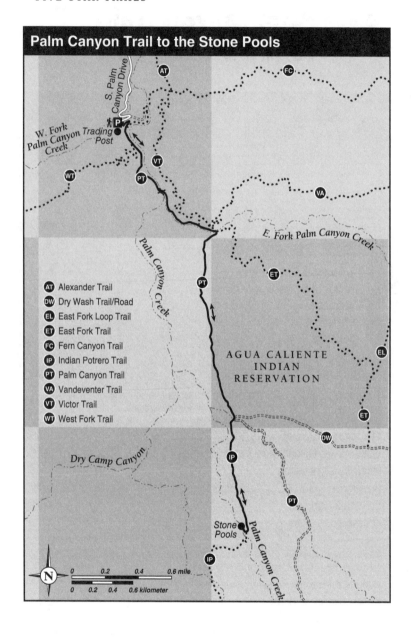

AT Alexander Trail
DW Dry Wash Trail/Road
EL East Fork Loop Trail
ET East Fork Trail
FC Fern Canyon Trail
IP Indian Potrero Trail
PT Palm Canyon Trail
VA Vandeventer Trail
VT Victor Trail
WT West Fork Trail

AGUA CALIENTE
INDIAN
RESERVATION

W. Fork Palm Canyon Creek
S. Palm Canyon Drive
Palm Canyon Trading Post
E. Fork Palm Canyon Creek
Palm Canyon Creek
Dry Camp Canyon
Stone Pools
Palm Canyon Creek

N

0   0.2   0.4   0.6 mile
0   0.2   0.4   0.6 kilometer

Overview

This out-and-back hike begins with a flat streamside stroll through fan palms and ancient rock mortars, then climbs past cactus scrub to expansive views of the desert and San Jacinto Mountains. Fifteen miles long, Palm Canyon Trail extends deep into the Indian Canyons, hooking up with several other dirt trails and fire roads. This hike stops at the Stone Pools, a striking cluster of rock gorges that beckon you to rest and frolic a bit before turning around. There is no shade after the first mile, so a hat and sunscreen are essential.

Route Details

Begin by descending to Palm Canyon via the concrete walkway just south of the Trading Post, a gift shop, refreshment stand, and information center for the Indian Canyons. Once home to the Agua Caliente band of Cahuilla Indians, Palm Canyon contains the largest naturally occurring stand of California fan palms in the United States. The first mile of this trail is shaded by a thick sea of fan palms and winds past a stream that can be lush and full after rains, but it's more of a trickle in late fall or in drought conditions. You'll also pass rock mortars that were used by the Agua Caliente band to grind fruits, seeds, and nuts 2,000 years ago. Much of the path is a mix of sand and rock, so sturdy shoes are a good idea.

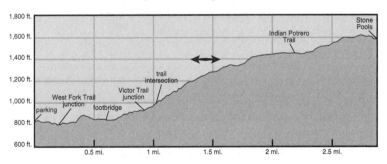

At 0.5 mile, you'll cross a small stream. Continue 0.25 mile through the palm jungle, bearing left at a small wooden post marked PALM CANYON. Continue another quarter-mile to another signed wooden post marking a junction. Here the Palm Canyon Trail continues straight, and the Victor Trail loops to the east and back to the Trading Post. With its moderate 300-foot elevation gain, the 3-mile round-trip Victor Trail is good for novice hikers or older children.

To continue to the Stone Pools, head south on Palm Canyon as it climbs uphill to a ridge that gives way to wide-open desert and canyon views. After 2 miles, you'll come to a trail junction. Dry Wash Trail, a dusty path favored by equestrians, is to your left (east), while the Palm Canyon and Indian Potrero Trails continue straight (south). Stay to the right on the Indian Potrero Trail for about 0.6 mile until you come to a sign for the Stone Pools. In a non-drought year, the pools will live up to their name with water flowing freely around boulders at the canyon bottom. But even if there is no water (as was the case during my last visit), it's still a cool and peaceful place to rest and re-energize before heading back on the dusty trail. My son had fun leaping around the boulders and exploring all the caves and nooks, and we had the whole place to ourselves.

End the hike back at the Trading Post, which sells ice-cold drinks, as well as maps, postcards, and Native American art and jewelry. On weekends, the park offers ranger-led 1-mile hikes that include talks about the area's human and natural history.

Directions

From southbound I-10, take Exit 111 and drive south 9.4 miles on CA 111 through downtown Palm Springs. Continue straight (south) on South Palm Canyon Drive for about 3 miles to the Indian Canyons toll gate, where you can pick up a map and pay the entrance fee. Follow the road south until it ends at the parking lot of the Trading Post.

Tahquitz Canyon Trail

SCENERY: ★ ★ ★
TRAIL CONDITION: ★ ★ ★
CHILDREN: ★ ★ ★
DIFFICULTY: ★ ★
SOLITUDE: ★ ★ ★

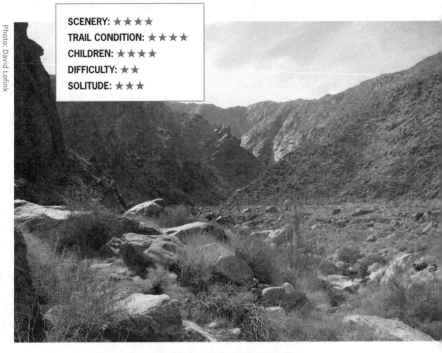

ROCKY HILLSIDES AND ANCIENT BOULDERS ALONG THE TRAIL

GPS TRAILHEAD COORDINATES: N33° 48.595' W116° 33.150'

DISTANCE & CONFIGURATION: 1.9-mile loop

HIKING TIME: 1 hour, 30 minutes

OUTSTANDING FEATURES: seasonal waterfalls, rock formations, Native American pictographs

ELEVATION GAIN: 300'

ACCESS: Open daily 7:30 a.m.–3:30 p.m. October–June, Friday–Sunday July–September. Admission: $12.50 per adult/$6 ages 12 and under.

MAPS: Detailed maps are available at the visitor center.

FACILITIES: Visitor center with restrooms, cold drinks, and gifts for sale

WHEELCHAIR ACCESS: None

COMMENTS: No pets or bikes on trails. Gates close at 5 p.m., and no vehicles are allowed in after 4 p.m.

CONTACTS: 714-323-6018, **tahquitzcanyon.com**

Tahquitz Canyon Trail

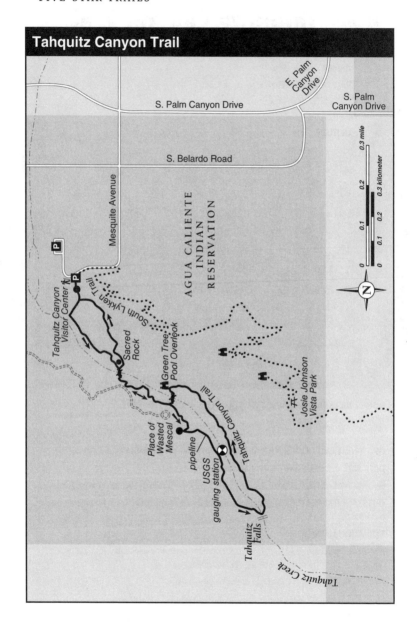

Overview

Framed by the San Jacinto Mountains to the west, this figure-eight hike follows Tahquitz Creek on a gradual ascent past ancient rocks and plants to a 60-foot-high waterfall. The admission fee seems a bit steep when there are so many good hikes in the area, but keep in mind that it goes to a good cause: maintaining the canyon's current pristine condition after years of abuse. It's a particularly fine hike in the spring when the falls and creek are robust with water.

Route Details

Tahquitz Canyon belongs to the Agua Caliente band of Cahuilla Indians and is listed in the National Register of Historic Places. Tahquitz comes from the name of an Indian shaman who was banished to the canyon when he abused his powers. The tribe believes his spirit still lives within the canyon walls and that he is searching for the souls of those who get too close to his lair. Squatters lived in the area for decades before the tribe kicked them out and spent four years cleaning up the graffiti and vandalism that was left behind. The canyon reopened for guided tours in 2001; now it allows visitors to take self-guided hikes on a 2-mile loop trail. (There are also regular guided

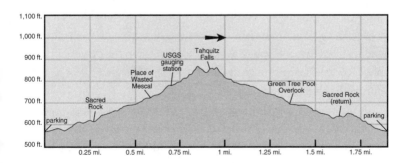

hikes by tribal rangers in season.) You will be cautioned to stay on the trails during your visit.

The trailhead begins just behind the visitor center, where you pay the fee and receive a map. Follow the rock-and-sand path southwest toward the mountains. An easy walk past creosote bush and barrel cactus gets you to your first sight: Sacred Rock, home of one of the oldest Cahuilla village sites. Stop and examine the painted prehistoric designs on the rock, then follow the path to the right, so you're on the right (west) side of the creek. Some of the other native plants to look for are desert apricot, white sage, Mormon tea, jojoba, and desert mistletoe.

At 0.6 mile, the path skirts a huge boulder, then reaches a fork. Stay to the right of the bridge; the left path also leads to Tahquitz Falls, but taking the westward route makes for a fun loop. Now the stream is to your left. Soon you'll come to a rusty gate and a water ditch on the right. This is known as the Place of Wasted Mescal and was used by the Cahuilla to bring drinking water from the canyon to the village. At about 0.8 mile, the trail skirts a long, thick water pipe on the right and moves closer to Tahquitz Creek, which is more of a trickle in summer. Follow the path up a series of natural rock steps and past a US Geological Survey gauging station, which was built in 1947 and is still monitored today. Continue heading southwest as the trail climbs toward the waterfall. At the 1-mile marker, the path hugs a sheer granite wall on the right, then comes to Tahquitz Falls, a lovely 60-foot-high waterfall that seems to flow from nowhere. Stop and rest here (even if you're not tired) and soak up the power of the place. (*Note:* During drought years, the waterfall may not flow at all during the summer and fall.)

From here the path loops around to the northeast and heads up, then down, a series of rocky steps. The creek is on your left. Soon you'll have great views of Palm Springs and Mount San Gorgonio straight ahead. Contemplate the massive rocks that cover the landscape, and take time to appreciate their pristine condition. It wasn't too long ago that the whole area was littered with graffiti and trash.

At 1.6 miles, you'll come to an overlook for Green Tree Pool, marked by a couple of large boulders: This is allegedly the site where a young Cahuilla woman was abducted and returned by Tahquitz himself.

Soon the trail curves left and crosses a small rock bridge. Just before reaching Sacred Rock again, you'll cross another small bridge, then meet up with the trail on which you started. Stay right to take the trail back to the visitor center (the path straight ahead is the way you already came). Piles of ancient dark-brown boulders line the hillside to your right as more views of Palm Springs and the Coachella Valley come into focus. Soon the path begins another gradual descent on wide rocky steps, with the visitor center ahead.

Although I enjoyed the peace and solitude of hiking Tahquitz Canyon by myself, I can also understand the appeal of taking a guided hike and learning more about the canyon's fascinating history. This is a convenient and fun hike for all levels of hikers, and it's easily reachable from downtown Palm Springs.

Nearby Attractions

Tahquitz Canyon is an easy 2-minute drive from the main drag of Palm Canyon Drive in Palm Springs. Reward yourself after your hike with burgers, fresh-squeezed lemonade, and coleslaw at the always-buzzing **Tyler's,** an iconic indoor/outdoor lunch spot at 149 S. Indian Canyon Dr. (**tylersburgers.com**).

Directions

From southbound I-10, take Exit 111 and drive south 9.4 miles on CA 111 through downtown Palm Springs. Continue straight (south) on South Palm Canyon Drive for about 2.5 miles. At West Mesquite Avenue, turn right and follow the signs to Tahquitz Canyon.

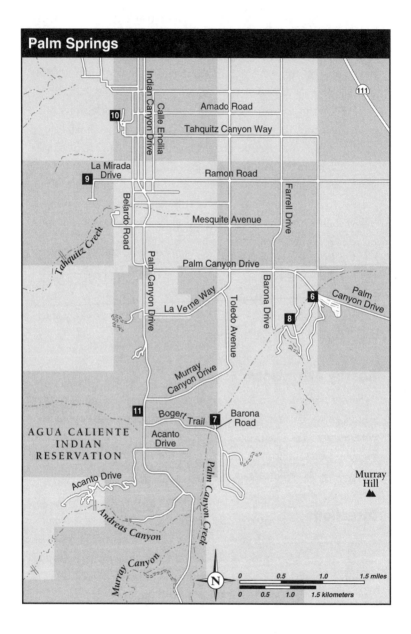

Palm Springs

Indian Canyon Drive

Calle Encilia

10

Amado Road

Tahquitz Canyon Way

La Mirada Drive

9

Ramon Road

Belardo Road

Farrell Drive

Tahquitz Creek

Mesquite Avenue

Palm Canyon Drive

Palm Canyon Drive

La Verne Way

Toledo Avenue

Barona Drive

6

Palm Canyon Drive

8

Murray Canyon Drive

11

Bogert Trail

7

Barona Road

AGUA CALIENTE INDIAN RESERVATION

Acanto Drive

Palm Canyon Creek

Murray Hill ▲

Acanto Drive

Andreas Canyon

Murray Canyon

N

| 0 | | 0.5 | | 1.0 | | 1.5 miles |

| 0 | | 0.5 | | 1.0 | | 1.5 kilometers |

111

Palm Springs

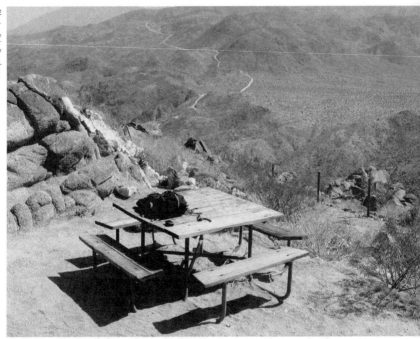

A PICNIC TABLE OFFERS SCENIC VIEWS FROM THE TOP OF MURRAY PEAK IN PALM SPRINGS. *(See Hike 7, page 52.)*

6 # Araby Trail

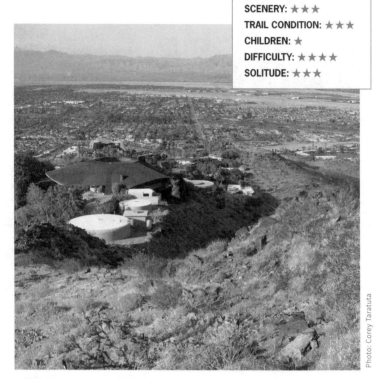

Photo: Corey Taratuta

A BIRD'S EYE VIEW OF THE FRANK LAUTNER–DESIGNED HOME ONCE OWNED BY BOB HOPE

GPS TRAILHEAD COORDINATES: N33° 47.847' W116° 30.584'

DISTANCE & CONFIGURATION: 3-mile out-and-back

HIKING TIME: 2–3 hours

HIGHLIGHTS: Desert and valley views, cactus scrub, Bob Hope's former house

ELEVATION GAIN: 1,300'

ACCESS: Trailhead open sunrise–sunset. Stay on the trail and heed the NO TRESPASSING signs of the nearby gated community.

MAPS: None

FACILITIES: Small parking area; no restrooms

WHEELCHAIR ACCESS: None

COMMENTS: Hats and sunscreen are a must for this shadeless hike.

CONTACTS: Palm Springs Bureau of Tourism, 760-778-8415, **visitpalmsprings.com**

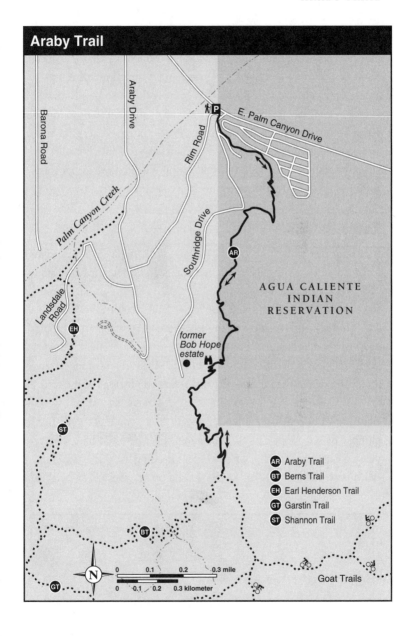

Araby Trail

Barona Road

Araby Drive

Palm Canyon Creek

Rim Road

Southridge Drive

P

E. Palm Canyon Drive

AR

AGUA CALIENTE
INDIAN
RESERVATION

former
Bob Hope
estate

Landsdale
Road

EH

ST

BT

GT

AR Araby Trail
BT Berns Trail
EH Earl Henderson Trail
GT Garstin Trail
ST Shannon Trail

Goat Trails

N

| 0 | 0.1 | 0.2 | 0.3 mile |

| 0 | 0.1 | 0.2 | 0.3 kilometer |

Overview

This hike begins outside an exclusive gated community that was once home to Bob Hope and Steve McQueen, and it turns into a strenuous ascent up shadeless switchbacks that come within a stone's throw of Hope's *Jetsons*-like former home. Locals call it "the trail to Bob Hope's house," but it also connects with other paths within the desert trail system, including the Garstin, Berns, and Clara Burgess Trails. Boasting an elevation gain of 1,300 feet, this hike is appreciated more for its good cardio workout and celebrity connection than for its attractive views.

Route Details

From the east end of the parking pullout, walk up paved Southridge Drive and look for the Palm Springs Trail sign on the left (east) side of the road. The narrow gravel-and-dirt path starts a gradual ascent toward the south. To the left you'll see (and hear) traffic from CA 111; to the right is a view of the mansions that sit behind the big gates you just left behind. From here on, most of the scenery is desert scrub and brown hillsides. It is best hiked in the early morning or late afternoon, when the hillsides provide shade on portions of the trail.

At 0.6 mile, you'll pass some PRIVATE PROPERTY signs on the right, and the trail curves left. If you look up, you'll get your first glimpse of Bob Hope's house, but don't linger here too long. Better views await. The trail dips briefly before heading back up the mountain via wide switchbacks. At the 1-mile point, you will be within

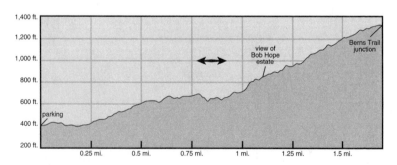

shouting distance of Bob Hope's house. The dome-shaped house, designed by architect John Lautner, is 25,000 square feet of glass and poured concrete. It has been called the "flying saucer house" and the "LAX terminal" because of its space-age appearance. (Hope died in 2003, and the house went on the market for $50 million in 2013. It was still for sale two years later, at a reduced price of $25 million.)

Continue past the house and its protective fence as the path meanders up the hillside. There is a paved street to the right that is part of the Southridge development, but heed the NO TRESPASSING signs and continue hiking along the Araby Trail. Soon you'll pass a few big boulders that are among the rare resting places on this narrow trail. From here you've got another half-mile ascent up wide switchbacks before you reach the mountain ridge. At 1.5 miles, you will come to an intersection and a sign for the Garstin and Berns trails, which form a single trail here that heads to the right. You can hook up with these trails and extend the hike or turn around and retrace your route to Southridge Drive.

Nearby Attractions

Hungry for more insights into the area's Hollywood and architectural history? **Palm Springs Modern Tours** (760-318-6118, **palmsprings moderntours.com**) leads visitors to historic neighborhoods and homes, including Araby Cove, and accompanies the driving tours with fun anecdotes about the architects, celebrities, and other assorted characters who lived and played here in the midcentury.

Directions

From downtown Palm Springs, follow Palm Canyon Drive (CA 111B) about 5 miles east toward Palm Desert. Make a right on Southridge Drive—if you pass Gene Autry Trail, you've gone too far east—and park at the turnout on the right (south) side of the road. Walk up the paved development road and look for the trailhead on the left-hand side; it begins about a quarter-mile below a locked gate.

Clara Burgess Trail

> SCENERY: ★ ★ ★
> TRAIL CONDITION: ★ ★ ★
> CHILDREN: ★ ★
> DIFFICULTY: ★ ★ ★ ★
> SOLITUDE: ★ ★ ★

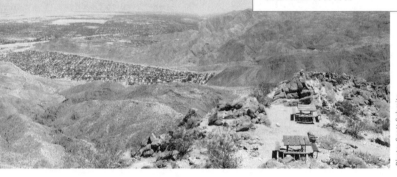

Photo: Scott Schmitz

PANORAMIC VIEWS OF THE COACHELLA VALLEY BECKON HIKERS TO THE TOP OF MURRAY HILL.

GPS COORDINATES: N33° 46.581' W116° 31.828'

DISTANCE & CONFIGURATION: 7.6-mile out-and-back

HIKING TIME: 3 hours, 30 minutes–4 hours

HIGHLIGHTS: Desert and valley views, solitude, cactus scrub

ELEVATION GAIN: 1,500'

ACCESS: Trailhead open sunrise–sunset

MAPS: None

FACILITIES: Street parking; no restrooms or water

WHEELCHAIR ACCESS: None

COMMENTS: Hats and sunscreen are a must for this shadeless hike.

CONTACTS: Palm Springs Bureau of Tourism, 760-778-8415, **visitpalmsprings.com**

Overview

This hike within the Palm Springs trail system begins with a strenuous switchback climb, then levels for a mile or so of easy walking before returning to a final hardy climb to the top of Murray Hill.

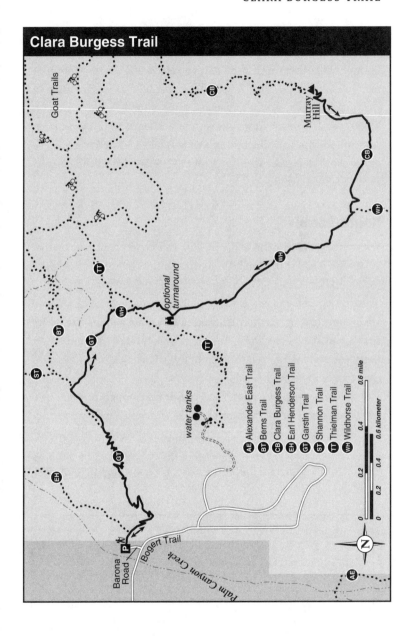

Clara Burgess Trail

Goat Trails

Murray Hill

CB

CB

WH

WH

TT

WH

BT

GT

ST

TT

optional turnaround

water tanks

GT

EH

Barona Road

P

Bogert Trail

Palm Canyon Creek

AE

AE Alexander East Trail
BT Berns Trail
CB Clara Burgess Trail
EH Earl Henderson Trail
GT Garstin Trail
ST Shannon Trail
TT Thielman Trail
WH Wildhorse Trail

N

0   0.2   0.4   0.6 mile

0   0.2   0.4   0.6 kilometer

It requires you to take two other trails, the Garstin and Wildhorse, which eventually link to the Clara Burgess Trail (named for a Palm Springs philanthropist). Ultimately, you arrive at a clearing with picnic tables and 360-degree views of the Coachella Valley. The path is well maintained and easy to navigate, with a total elevation gain of 1,500 feet. It's a good idea to wear sturdy shoes and bring a hiking companion with you. The last mile of this hike is closed from January to June each year, which is lambing season for the endangered Peninsular bighorn sheep.

Route Details

The trail begins at the end of Barona Road off Bogert Trail. Park on the street and look for the trailhead to the right of the road barrier that overlooks Palm Canyon Wash. The path, composed of packed dirt and small rocks, immediately climbs uphill via wide switchbacks. Soon you'll come to a signpost for Smoketree Mountain and the Shannon, Araby, and Wildhorse Trails. Continue straight ahead toward these trails; you still have another 2 miles of robust hiking before you reach the Clara Burgess Trail.

The residential development you drove through to reach the trailhead is now below you on the right. Its landscaped yards and swimming pools are quite a contrast to the scrub-covered hillsides toward which you're heading. After another 100 yards or so, you will reach another signpost; follow the Garstin Trail straight ahead. The

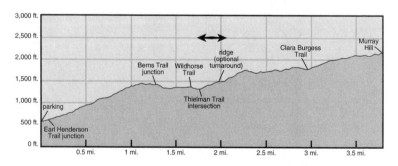

Earl Henderson Trail branches left and continues on a rugged northeast route to the edge of East Palm Canyon Drive. The Garstin Trail keeps its gradual ascent via wide switchbacks. At the half-mile marker, the trail skirts a small clearing with views of Palm Springs and a sign that says dogs prohibited beyond this point. This is a critical habitat for endangered Peninsular bighorn sheep, and wildlife experts fear that the presence of dogs may cause the sheep to flee the area.

From here, continue another half-mile to an unmarked fork; you want to follow the trail to the right and up the hill. Palm Springs and the entire Coachella Valley come into view and weave in and out of sight the rest of the way up the mountain. After passing another rocky clearing, you will come to a signpost at 1.2 miles. Take the trail to the right toward the Garstin Trail. The trail to the left leads to Berns Trail, a connector trail that links with the Araby Trail. Now you'll really start to feel the solitude and total escape that characterizes this hike. I didn't see a single person when I hiked this trail on a Saturday afternoon in mid-November. It was a hot day, but the hillsides cast shadows on much of the trail, making it a pleasant late-afternoon excursion.

At 1.5 miles, the trail forks again; heed the wooden signpost that says TRAIL and continue straight on an eastern route. Pass a large wood sign that says GARSTIN TRAIL; head straight, toward the sign for the Clara Burgess Trail.

At this point, the trail begins to climb again and turns to loose gravel for a bit, then goes back to packed dirt. You'll catch glimpses of the residential development again to your right, but it will seem like you're a world away.

At 2.2 miles, you will come to a clearing with a couple of big rocks overlooking the valley. This is a good place to stop and rest before continuing to Murray Hill; it's also a good turnaround point for those who prefer a shorter hike or those who worry about making it back to the trailhead before the sun sets.

To continue to the Clara Burgess Trail, head straight (southeast) along the mountain ridge. From here the trail levels for an easy half-mile before reaching the Clara Burgess Trailhead and starting its final ascent to Murray Hill. At 3 miles, you'll come to a sign marking the Clara Burgess Trailhead. The White Horse Trail continues to the right and eventually connects with Fern Canyon Trail and the Indian Canyons. You want to continue straight and follow the Clara Burgess east over the hillside. The views keep getting better and better as you walk. You're at an elevation of about 2,000 feet at this point, and you can see the entire Coachella Valley, as well as the Little San Bernardino Mountains to the north.

At 3.4 miles, Murray Hill comes into view to the east. Another 0.4 miles of strenuous switchbacking brings you to the top. Once you arrive, you'll see why this hike is worth every drop of sweat. The panoramic mountain and valley views are breathtaking. Have some water and a snack at one of the two picnic tables at the top before heading back down the mountain. The hike back to Bogert Trail isn't likely to take as long because it is mostly downhill.

Directions

From southbound I-10, take CA 111 south 9.4 miles through downtown Palm Springs. Merge right onto South Palm Canyon Drive and continue about 4.75 miles to Bogert Trail, a paved residential street. Make a left and follow Bogert about 0.9 mile, just past the bridge that crosses the wash. Make a left on Barona Road, the first road after the wash, and park at the end. The unmarked trailhead is to the right.

8 # Earl Henderson Trail

SCENERY: ★ ★ ★ ★
TRAIL CONDITION: ★ ★ ★
CHILDREN: ★ ★
DIFFICULTY: ★ ★ ★
SOLITUDE: ★ ★ ★ ★

Photo: Eric Forsberg

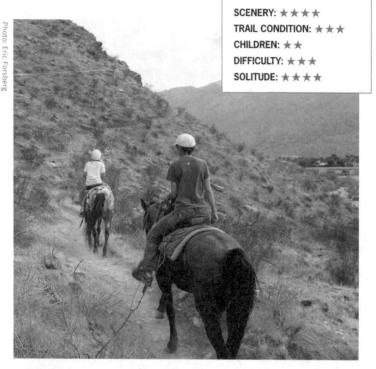

EQUESTRIANS SHARE THE EARL HENDERSON TRAIL WITH BACKCOUNTRY HIKERS.

GPS TRAILHEAD COORDINATES: N33° 47.609' W116° 30.846'

DISTANCE & CONFIGURATION: 4-mile out-and-back

HIKING TIME: 2 hours

HIGHLIGHTS: Desert and valley views, solitude, desert vegetation

ELEVATION GAIN: 300'

ACCESS: Trailhead open sunrise–sunset

MAPS: None

FACILITIES: Street parking; no restrooms or water

WHEELCHAIR ACCESS: None

COMMENTS: Hats and sunscreen are a must for this shadeless hike.

CONTACTS: Palm Springs Bureau of Tourism, 760-778-8415, **visitpalmsprings.com**

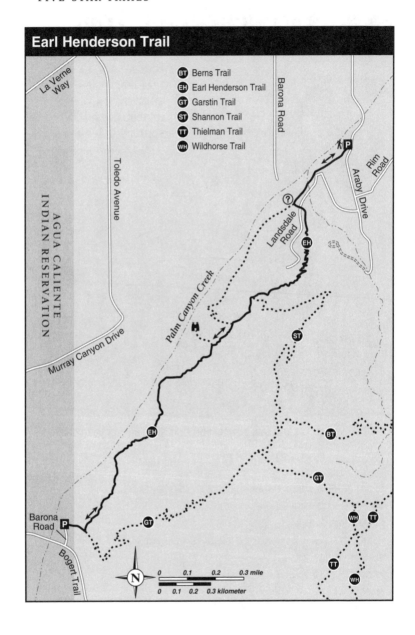

Earl Henderson Trail

BT Berns Trail
EH Earl Henderson Trail
GT Garstin Trail
ST Shannon Trail
TT Thielman Trail
WH Wildhorse Trail

Overview

Named for local equestrian Earl Henderson, this unassuming horse and hiking trail begins in a desert-wash landscape, then zigzags around a mountainside to connect with other trails in the Palm Springs trail system. It's not the most dazzling of the Palm Springs trails, but it's a reliable, less strenuous alternative to the nearby Araby Trail. It has a moderate elevation gain and is popular with dog walkers and horseback riders from nearby Smoketree Ranch.

OPTION The trail can also be accessed from Bogert Trail off South Palm Canyon Drive at the same trailhead that leads to the Garstin and Clara Burgess Trails. Follow South Palm Canyon Trail to Bogert Trail and turn left. After crossing a small bridge, turn left and park at the end of the street. Arrange for a friend to pick you up at Araby Drive, or retrace your route to Bogert Trail.

Route Details

From the parking pullout, walk across the street to the desert wash and begin hiking south amid the creosote bushes and tumbleweed. There is no marked trail for the first half-mile of this hike; just follow the sandy wash until you come to a trail junction for the Henderson, Berns, Garstin, Shannon, and Palm Springs Trails. (*Note:*

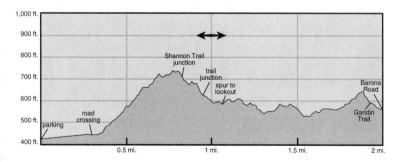

"Henderson" refers to the Earl Henderson Trail, not the Randall Henderson Trail, which is off CA 74 in Palm Desert and is profiled in Hike 19.) Veer left on the Henderson Trail and cross a paved road to get to the actual trailhead. The other trails continue straight (south) toward a mountain. At 0.6 mile, you'll come to a large metal sign marking the entrance to the Earl Henderson Trail. Now you're on a singletrack, sand-and-rock trail surrounded by brown hillsides and moving farther away from busy Palm Canyon Drive and its developments. After a short distance, the path begins to switchback up the mountain. The next quarter-mile is the steepest part of the hike.

At 0.85 mile, you'll come to a faded sign that says, "1968: This trail maintained for your riding and hiking pleasure in memory of Earl Henderson and Lucky." From here the path heads down a short hill, then levels and hugs the hillside for the rest of the way. Development creeps back into view in the distance to the right, but you will feel far removed from it all. The canyon wash also comes back into view on the west. At about 1 mile, you will pass a small sign for the Palm Springs Trail, then a narrow trail on the right that heads west about a quarter-mile to a small lookout. Continue straight on the Earl Henderson Trail. At 1.75 miles, the trail heads downhill toward the canyon wash, then back up the mountain in a gradual ascent toward a trail junction that overlooks southern Palm Springs and the San Jacinto Mountains. From here you have three options: retrace your steps back to Araby Drive; continue your hike by taking the Garstin Trail southeast into the mountains; or take the path to the west down the hill toward Bogert Trail and have someone pick you up there, making the hike 2 miles instead of 4.

Nearby Attractions

One of the oldest and finest resorts in Palm Springs is a stone's throw from this trail. **Smoke Tree Ranch** (800-787-3922, **smoketreeranch.com**) has been accommodating guests like Walt Disney and Diane Keaton since the mid-1930s. Its guest ranch, simple cottages, and landscaped desert scenery are straight out of an old western, and it prides itself on providing a private, genteel experience complete with three meals a day and recreational activities like golf and tennis. Studio cottages start at $400 per night. The ranch is closed during the summer.

Directions

From downtown Palm Springs, follow Palm Canyon Drive (CA 111B) about 4.7 miles east toward Palm Desert. At South Araby Drive, turn right (south), drive about 0.6 mile, and look for an unpaved parking pullout on the left.

North Lykken Trail

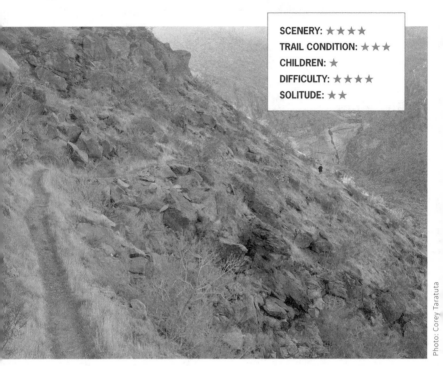

SCENERY: ★ ★ ★ ★
TRAIL CONDITION: ★ ★ ★
CHILDREN: ★
DIFFICULTY: ★ ★ ★ ★
SOLITUDE: ★ ★

Photo: Corey Taratuta

**SOLITUDE AND STRIKING MOUNTAIN-AND-DESERT VIEWS MARK THE
NORTH LYKKEN TRAIL.**

GPS TRAILHEAD COORDINATES: N33° 48.964' W116° 33.286' (trailhead),
N33° 50.767' W116° 33.737' (Cielo Drive shuttle)

DISTANCE & CONFIGURATION: 3-mile out-and-back or 4.5-mile point-to-point with shuttle

HIKING TIME: 2 hours, 30 minutes–3 hours, 30 minutes

OUTSTANDING FEATURES: desert vegetation, ancient rock formations, views of
Palm Springs and the Coachella Valley

ELEVATION GAIN: 800'

ACCESS: Trailhead open sunrise–sunset

MAPS: At trailhead kiosk

FACILITIES: Street parking; no restrooms or water

WHEELCHAIR ACCESS: None

COMMENTS: Hats and sunscreen are a must for this shadeless hike.

CONTACTS: Palm Springs Bureau of Tourism, 760-778-8415, **visitpalmsprings.com**

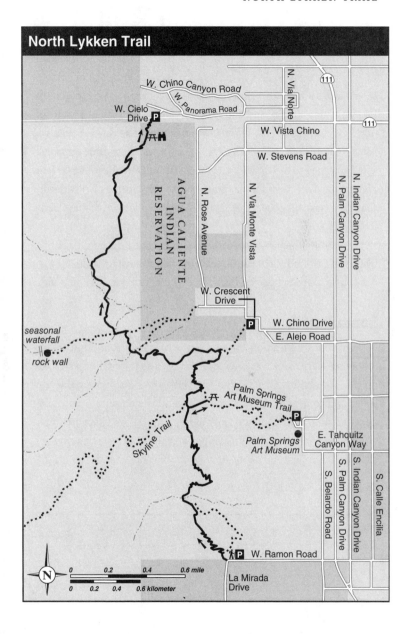

North Lykken Trail

Overview

The North Lykken Trail is the north half of the 9.5-mile Carl Lykken Trail, which weaves along a series of mountain ridges above downtown Palm Springs. This shuttle hike begins at the west end of Ramon Road in Palm Springs and ends at Cielo Drive, off Vista Chino Road, north of downtown. It's more strenuous and less crowded than the south half of the Carl Lykken Trail (known widely as the South Lykken Trail) (see page 70), with a total elevation gain of about 800 feet, and it links with two popular trails—the Palm Springs Art Museum Trail (see next hike) and the Skyline Trail, also known as the Cactus to Clouds Trail.

OPTION This can also be a moderate 3-mile out-and-back hike by turning around at the picnic-table overlook above the Palm Springs Art Museum, then heading back the way you came to Ramon Road.

Route Details

Look for the trailhead on the right (north) side of Ramon Road and follow the narrow rock-and-sand path north as it switchbacks up the hillside for about 0.3 mile. You will pass a signpost where the trail levels and continues to curve north around the mountain ridge. The next 0.5 mile is a moderate walk along a mountain ridge accompanied by terrific views of Palm Springs and the Coachella Valley to the east. At 0.8 mile, the trail begins to climb again, then levels until it

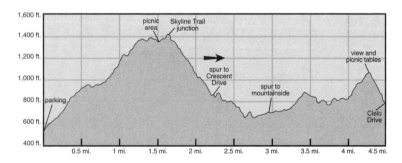

reaches a turnoff for the Palm Springs Art Museum Trail on the right. Continue straight to stay on the Lykken Trail, or take the Museum Trail 0.2 mile to a clearing with picnic tables. Here you can have a snack and enjoy the view before reconnecting with the Lykken Trail. This is a good turnaround point for a 3-mile out-and-back hike.

To continue the shuttle hike, head northwest at the trail split and follow the Lykken Trail around the mountain as it begins a gradual descent into Chino Canyon. After walking about 1.3 miles from the trail split, you will come to an unsigned fork. Bear right; the left trail heads west for about 0.5 mile and dead-ends at a mountainside popular with rock climbers. Follow the trail across a canyon wash, then up a hillside to a clearing with picnic tables and another scenic viewpoint. From here it's a short but very steep hike down the side of the hillside to Cielo Drive. Wear sturdy hiking shoes and beware of loose gravel here. If you haven't left a second car or arranged for a pickup, turn back at the picnic tables and retrace your route to Ramon Road and the southern trailhead.

Nearby Attractions

See next hike.

Directions

From southbound I-10, take Exit 111 and drive south 9.4 miles on CA 111 through downtown Palm Springs. Continue straight (south) on South Palm Canyon Drive about 2 miles; at West Ramon Road, turn right and continue to the end. Park on the street.

To leave a shuttle car, follow the directions above through the first sentence. Turn right (west) off South Palm Canyon Drive onto West Vista Chino, then turn right (north) on North Via Norte and left on West Chino Canyon Road. At the T-intersection, bear left on West Panorama Road; then, at the fork in the road, bear left on West Cielo Drive and follow it to the end.

Palm Springs Art Museum Trail

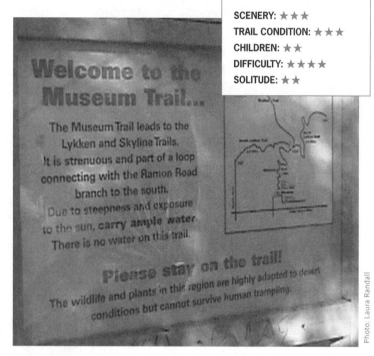

SCENERY: ★ ★ ★
TRAIL CONDITION: ★ ★ ★
CHILDREN: ★ ★
DIFFICULTY: ★ ★ ★ ★
SOLITUDE: ★ ★

Welcome to the Museum Trail...

The Museum Trail leads to the Lykken and Skyline Trails. It is strenuous and part of a loop connecting with the Ramon Road branch to the south. Due to steepness and exposure to the sun, carry ample water. There is no water on this trail.

Please stay on the trail!

The wildlife and plants in this region are highly adapted to desert conditions but cannot survive human trampling.

Photo: Laura Randall

A SIGN AT THE START OF THE ART MUSEUM TRAIL WARNS HIKERS TO BE PREPARED FOR A STEEP UPHILL TREK.

GPS TRAILHEAD COORDINATES: N33° 49.529' W116° 32.946'

DISTANCE & CONFIGURATION: 2-mile out-and-back

HIKING TIME: 1 hour

HIGHLIGHTS: Steep, rocky hillside; cactus and desert scrub; city and valley views

ELEVATION GAIN: 850'

ACCESS: Trailhead open sunrise–sunset

MAPS: At trailhead kiosk

FACILITIES: Free parking; no restrooms or water

WHEELCHAIR ACCESS: None

COMMENTS: Hats and sunscreen are a must for this shadeless hike.

CONTACTS: Palm Springs Bureau of Tourism, 760-778-8415, **visitpalmsprings.com**

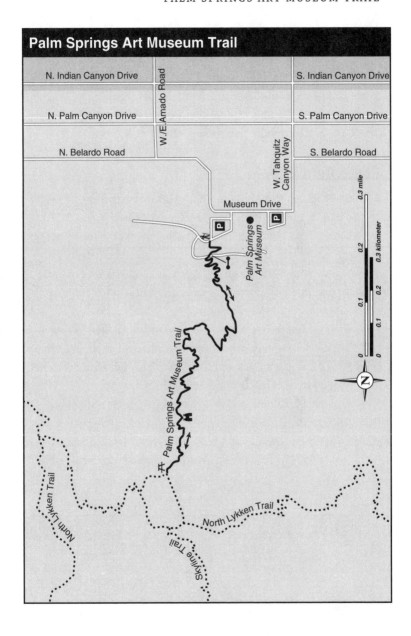

Palm Springs Art Museum Trail

N. Indian Canyon Drive

S. Indian Canyon Drive

W./E. Amado Road

N. Palm Canyon Drive

S. Palm Canyon Drive

N. Belardo Road

S. Belardo Road

W. Tahquitz Canyon Way

Museum Drive

Palm Springs Art Museum

Palm Springs Art Museum Trail

North Lykken Trail

North Lykken Trail

Skyline Trail

Overview

This popular hike begins near downtown Palm Springs and criss-crosses the mountainside, gaining 850 feet in elevation in just 1 mile. It links with the North and South Lykken Trails, as well as the very challenging Skyline Trail (also known as the Cactus to Clouds Trail), a relentless uphill climb to San Jacinto Peak.

Route Details

This hike is called the Museum Trail because it begins at the edge of the parking lot for the Palm Springs Art Museum, just off the town's main drag. Look for a map and sign that says welcome to the museum trail at the north end of the lot. There is no shade along the trail; water and sunscreen are essential. Locals use this cardio-friendly trail as an outdoor gym, so expect to see a fair number of other hikers, especially on weekends.

The trail immediately begins to wind uphill, flanked by a hand-rail on one side and piles of rocks on the other. Soon you'll reach a private road and gate to your left; cross the road and get back on the trail as it continues its ascent of the rocky hillside.

At about 0.75 mile, you will come to a clearing with views of Palm Springs and the distant mountains. From here the trail heads west toward the rocky hills and away from civilization. It levels for a bit before making its final brief ascent to a clearing with picnic tables

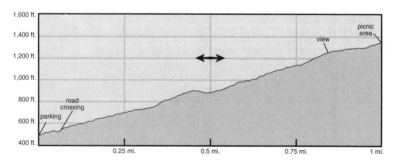

and more fine views of the valley. This marks the end of the Museum Trail. It's a good place to rest before heading back down the mountain.

You can also access the North Lykken Trail from this point, though you hit it right in the middle. To pick up the south half of the North Lykken Trail, head north briefly before veering south, and then follow a gradual descent down the hillside to the west end of Ramon Road. (See pages 62 and 70 for more details on the Lykken trails).

Nearby Attractions

This trail is within easy walking distance of downtown Palm Springs and its vibrant collection of shops and restaurants. There's even a lodging option that boasts direct access to the Museum Trail: **Colony 29 (colony29.com)** is a complex of six Spanish-style homes that can be rented out for vacations and events. A private trail on the property links with the public trail system.

Before tackling this hike, consider checking out the **Palm Springs Art Museum** (101 Museum Dr.; 760-322-4800, **psmuseum.org**), an excellent community hub with a modern-art collection, rotating exhibits, and a theater. It's so close, you won't even need to move your car.

Directions

From southbound I-10, take Exit 111 and drive south 9.4 miles on CA 111 through downtown Palm Springs. Continue straight (south) on North Palm Canyon Drive about 1.5 miles. Turn right on West Tahquitz Canyon Way, then make a right on Museum Drive. Park at the north end of the lot near the trail sign.

South Lykken Trail

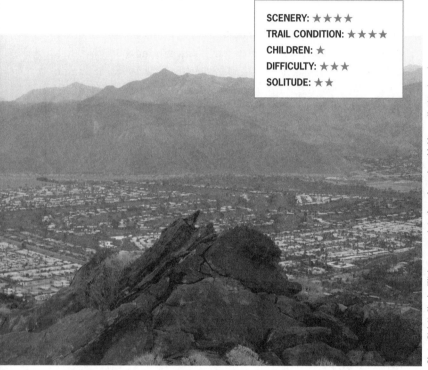

SCENERY: ★ ★ ★ ★
TRAIL CONDITION: ★ ★ ★ ★
CHILDREN: ★
DIFFICULTY: ★ ★ ★
SOLITUDE: ★ ★

LOOKING DOWN ON PALM SPRINGS FROM THE SOUTH LYKKEN TRAIL

GPS TRAILHEAD COORDINATES: N33° 46.723' W116° 32.715' (trailhead),
N33° 48.514› W116° 33.103' (Mesquite Avenue shuttle)

DISTANCE & CONFIGURATION: 2-mile out-and-back or 4.7-mile point-to-point with shuttle

HIKING TIME: 2 hours, 15 minutes–3 hours

HIGHLIGHTS: Desert and valley views, rocky hillsides

ELEVATION GAIN: 900'

ACCESS: Trailhead open sunrise–sunset

MAPS: At trailhead kiosk

FACILITIES: Free parking; no restrooms or water

WHEELCHAIR ACCESS: None

COMMENTS: Hats and sunscreen are a must for this shadeless hike.

CONTACTS: Palm Springs Bureau of Tourism, 760-778-8415, **visitpalmsprings.com**

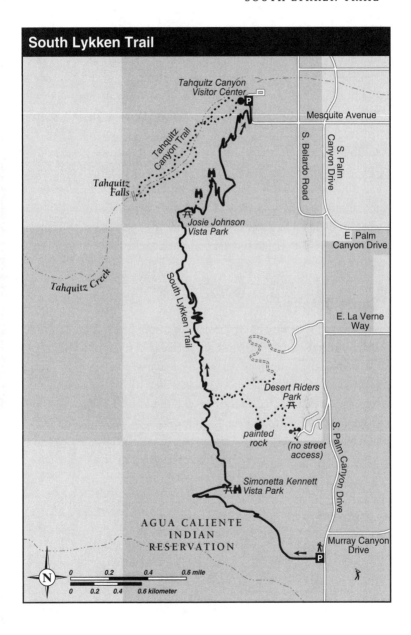

South Lykken Trail

Tahquitz Canyon
Visitor Center

Mesquite Avenue

Tahquitz
Canyon Trail

S. Belardo Road

S. Palm
Canyon Drive

Tahquitz
Falls

Josie Johnson
Vista Park

E. Palm
Canyon Drive

Tahquitz Creek

South Lykken Trail

E. La Verne
Way

Desert Riders
Park

painted
rock

(no street
access)

S. Palm Canyon Drive

Simonetta Kennett
Vista Park

AGUA CALIENTE
INDIAN
RESERVATION

Murray Canyon
Drive

N

0   0.2   0.4   0.6 mile

0   0.2   0.4   0.6 kilometer

Overview

The South Lykken Trail is the south half of the 9.5-mile Carl Lykken Trail, which weaves along a series of mountain ridges above downtown Palm Springs. The north and south trails are separated by Tahquitz Canyon, so you can't easily do them as one hike. The South Lykken Trail is a terrific moderate hike featuring panoramic views of the desert valley and a bird's-eye view of Tahquitz Canyon's waterfalls and rock formations. This shuttle hike begins at the south end, follows the trail up a moderately steep hillside, then winds along the mountain ridge past a couple of viewpoints before taking you back down into Tahquitz Canyon at Mesquite Avenue. Expect to see at least a handful of hikers and dogs on this popular trail on any given day of the week.

Route Details

Begin by walking west along the dirt road from South Palm Canyon Drive. After about 0.3 mile, the trail narrows and starts to switchback up the hillside to the right. A gradual climb over the next 0.75 mile takes you deeper into the rocky hillsides. You will pass a metal sign for the Carl Lykken Trail on the way up. After about 1 mile, you come to a viewpoint with a few picnic tables and a sign for Simonetta Kennett Vista Park. This is a good place to pause for a few minutes and admire the gorgeous views of the Coachella Valley to the east. It's also

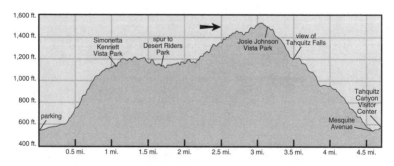

a turnaround point for a moderate 2-mile hike. For the shuttle hike, continue heading north on the trail as it snakes along the mountain ridge. After about 1.7 miles, you'll come to a trail split marked by a small pile of rocks, or cairn. From here, it's a short walk east on the spur trail to Desert Riders Park, a clearing with picnic tables and valley vistas.

To continue on to the shuttle hike, return to the Lykken Trail and continue following it northwest along the rocky mountain ridge. Views of Palm Springs and beyond accompany you for the rest of the hike to the trail's north terminus. After another 0.5 mile of walking, you'll come to another trail split—stay left and continue north on the Carl Lykken Trail. Three miles in, you'll come to another wide clearing with picnic tables, known as Josie Johnson Vista Park. This is your last chance to rest and soak up the beautiful views before heading back down the hillside to Mesquite Avenue. There are usually a few people relaxing here with their dogs or enjoying a picnic lunch. Hikers who haven't arranged for a shuttle pickup at Mesquite Avenue can turn around here and retrace their route to the Murray Canyon trailhead.

From the picnic tables, the trail winds east briefly before turning north toward Tahquitz Canyon. At about 3.4 miles, be sure to look left for an awesome view of the seasonal waterfall in Tahquitz Canyon (if it's summer, you might not see much). From here the trail heads east, then north again for another 1.5 miles before ending at the driveway for the Tahquitz Canyon Visitor Center. Parking is allowed on Mesquite Avenue, west of South Palm Canyon Drive.

Nearby Activities

Moorten Botanical Garden is located at 1701 S. Palm Canyon Dr., between the two access points for the South Lykken Trail (760-327-6555, **moortenbotanicalgarden.com**). Run by the same family since 1938, it's a peaceful oasis studded with thousands of species of rare and common desert plants, as well as rocks, crystals, and gold-mine artifacts. Tours are available, or you can wander around on your own.

There's a small admission fee ($4 adults, $2 kids 5–15) and a nursery that sells plants. It's closed Wednesdays year-round and operates Friday–Sunday only in summer.

Directions

From southbound I-10, take Exit 111 and drive south 9.4 miles on CA 111 through downtown Palm Springs. Continue straight (south) on South Palm Canyon Drive about 4.5 miles to just beyond Murray Canyon Drive. The trail begins on the right side of the street, just after the housing and condominium complexes give way to wide open fields. Park on Palm Canyon Drive, across from the golf course.

To leave a shuttle car, follow the directions above through the first sentence. Continue straight (south) on South Palm Canyon Drive for about 2.5 miles; at West Mesquite Avenue, turn right and follow the signs to Tahquitz Canyon.

THE GARSTIN TRAIL EVENTUALLY CONNECTS TO THE CLARA BURGESS TRAIL (HIKE 7), WHILE THE EARL HENDERSON TRAIL (HIKE 8) BRANCHES OFF TO THE NORTHEAST.

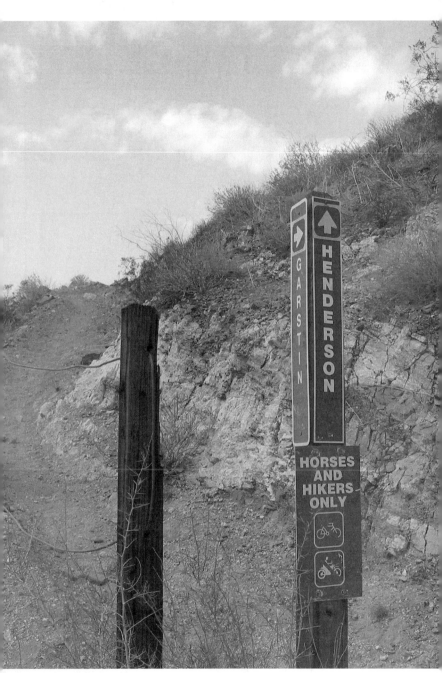

Photo: Eric Forsberg

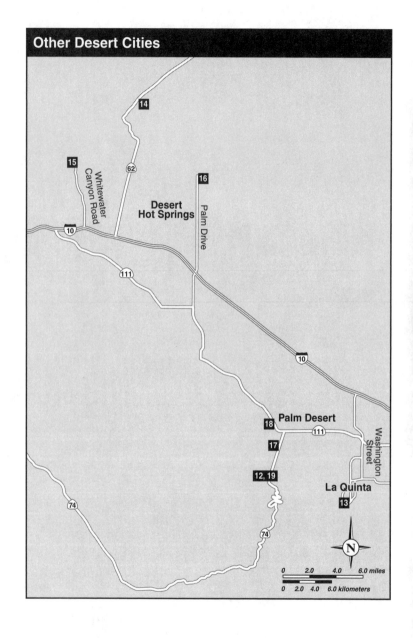

Other Desert Cities

14

15

62

Whitewater Canyon Road

16

Desert Hot Springs

Palm Drive

10

111

10

Palm Desert

18

111

17

Washington Street

12, 19

74

La Quinta

13

74

N

| 0 | 2.0 | 4.0 | 6.0 miles |
| 0 | 2.0 | 4.0 | 6.0 kilometers |

Other Desert Cities

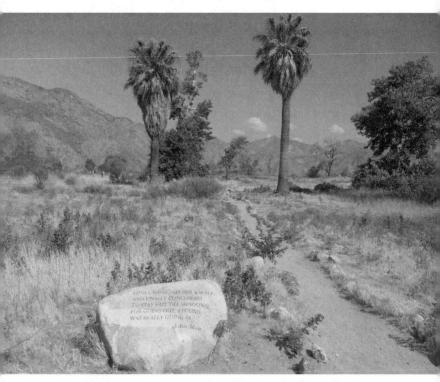

A JOHN MUIR QUOTE WELCOMES HIKERS TO THE CANYON VIEW TRAIL IN
WHITEWATER PRESERVE. *(See Hike 15, page 91.)*   Photo: Laura Randall

Art Smith Trail, Palm Desert

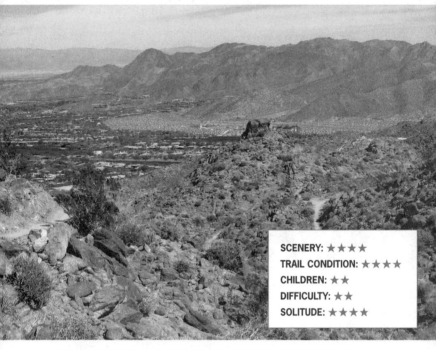

SCENERY: ★ ★ ★ ★
TRAIL CONDITION: ★ ★ ★ ★
CHILDREN: ★ ★
DIFFICULTY: ★ ★
SOLITUDE: ★ ★ ★ ★

**A VIEWPOINT ALONG THE ART SMITH TRAIL OVERLOOKS THE CITY OF
PALM DESERT AND BEYOND.** Photo: Eric Forsberg

GPS TRAILHEAD COORDINATES: N33° 40.138' W116° 24.615'

DISTANCE & CONFIGURATION: 6-mile out-and-back

HIKING TIME: 3–4 hours

HIGHLIGHTS: Palm groves, rock formations, panoramic views, bighorn sheep habitat

ELEVATION GAIN: 1,500'

ACCESS: Trailhead open sunrise–sunset

MAPS: None

FACILITIES: Free parking; no restrooms or water

WHEELCHAIR ACCESS: None

COMMENTS: Hats and sunscreen are a must for this shadeless hike.

CONTACTS: Palm Desert Visitor Center, 760-568-1441 or 800-873-2428,
palm-desert.org; Bureau of Land Management, 760-862-9984

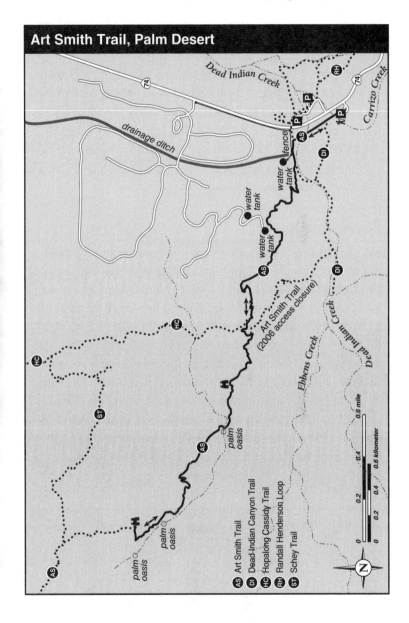

Art Smith Trail, Palm Desert

Dead Indian Creek

Carrizo Creek

drainage ditch

water fence
water tank
water tank
water tank

Art Smith Trail
(2006 access closure)

Ebbens Creek

Dead Indian Creek

palm oasis

palm oasis

palm oasis

0.6 mile
0.2   0.4
0   0.6 kilometer
0   0.2   0.4

AS Art Smith Trail
DI Dead-Indian Canyon Trail
HC Hopalong Cassidy Trail
RH Randall Henderson Loop
ST Schey Trail

Overview

Named after a local trail builder, this well-maintained trail is a long-time favorite of Palm Springs hikers and equestrians. It begins just off CA 74 in Palm Desert and switchbacks up a hillside before leveling and meandering for several miles past a series of palm oases and views of the Coachella Valley. It totals 6 miles out-and-back, but many day hikers take it to the second palm oasis or to Magnesia Springs Canyon, and then they turn back before the trail ends at Dunn Road, a vehicle-restricted road that leads to Cathedral City.

Route Details

Look for the trailhead at the far north corner of the parking lot. You will see a sign for the Art Smith Trail and a map of the Palm Springs area trail system. Begin walking north past the sign along the sandy wash. After 100 yards or so, you will come to a sign indicating that Dead Indian Canyon, a 3-mile out-and-back trail, is closed January 1– September 30. To pick up the Art Smith Trail, follow the base of the concrete drainage ditch, which is to the right of the sign, north along the wash. After a short walk, look for a water tank that sits beyond a chain-link fence with a gate. Make a sharp left just before the gate and follow the south side of the fence west toward the hillside. There is no real trail at this point; you are just walking across a wash of cracked, layered mud that has dried in stages. After 0.4 mile, look for a sign-post and a narrow dirt trail winding up the hillside just beyond it.

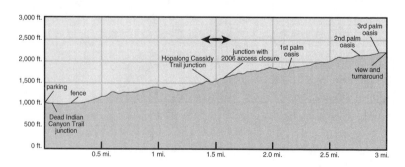

Follow the trail up the hill past desert lavender, sage, creosote bush, and barrel and cholla cactus. You can still see and hear traffic from CA 74 as you ascend, but every step gets you farther away from civilization. At 0.7 mile, the path levels and passes a small clearing marked by rock formations; this is a good spot for kids to explore, though they won't have much patience for the remaining shadeless 7 miles of this trail. From here it dips north into the canyon and provides views of the strangely green Bighorn Golf Club to the northeast. The trail continues for the next mile in easy switchbacks along the mountain ridge, past a few small boulder-strewn viewpoints overlooking the valley. You will begin to see more cacti, aloe, and other desert plants on either side of the trail.

At 1.5 miles, the Art Smith Trail connects with the 8-mile Hopalong Cassidy Trail, a relatively recent addition to the desert hiking system that leads to Homme-Adams Park in Palm Desert and the Mirage Trail in Rancho Mirage. Continue straight on Art Smith (the Hopalong Cassidy Trail veers right) as it follows the mountain ridge west. At about 2 miles, the trail crosses a flat clearing dotted with rock formations, then ascends a small hillside to a view of a small California fan-palm oasis. Follow the trail to the right of the palms, then look for an unsigned post and go left up a short, steep hill. Continue another 0.5 mile along a wide, sandy trail to a series of three more palm groves and fine views of the valley framed by rocky hillsides. At about 3 miles, you will reach a small clearing with boulders for sitting and more great views of the valley. This is a good turnaround point for those looking for a short day hike. Or you may continue another 2.2 miles to Magnesia Springs Canyon, home to another shady palm oasis that makes a good spot to stop for lunch. From Magnesia Springs Canyon, the Art Smith Trail winds northwest until it ends at Dunn Road, a no-vehicles road that links with the Hahn Buena Vista and Vandeventer Trails, two strenuous trails popular with mountain bikers within the Indian Canyons.

Nearby Attractions

The **Palm Desert Visitor Center** (73-470 El Paseo) has good hiking maps of the area and is a reliable source for updates on trail conditions and reroutes; it's open Monday–Saturday from 10 a.m. to 6 p.m. Also nearby is a satellite branch of the **Palm Springs Art Museum** (72-567 Highway 111, in the visitor center's previous headquarters; 760-346-5600, **psmuseum.org/palm-desert**). Also known as The Galen, it has rotating exhibits and a modern sculpture garden that's free and open to the public year-round. Its natural rock benches make a lovely place to rest weary bones after a hike.

Directions

From Palm Canyon Drive (CA 111) in Palm Desert, turn south on Pines to Palms Highway (CA 74). After about 4 miles, look for the small Art Smith Trail parking lot on the right, just past the visitor center for the Santa Rosa and San Jacinto Mountains National Monument.

13

Bear Creek Canyon Oasis, La Quinta

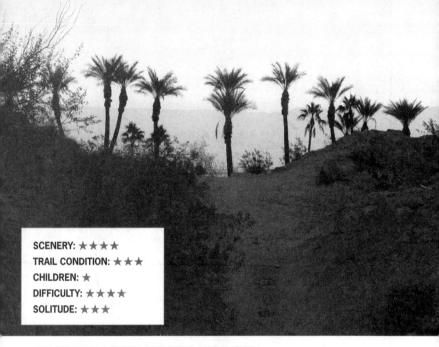

SCENERY: ★★★★
TRAIL CONDITION: ★★★
CHILDREN: ★
DIFFICULTY: ★★★★
SOLITUDE: ★★★

THIS PALM OASIS AWAITS AT THE END OF THE TRAIL. Photo: Laura Randall

GPS TRAILHEAD COORDINATES: N33° 38.922' W116° 19.039'

DISTANCE & CONFIGURATION: 9-mile out-and-back

HIKING TIME: 5.5–6 hours

HIGHLIGHTS: Cactus and desert scrub; rocky hillsides; sweeping city, valley, and mountain views

ELEVATION GAIN: 2,200'

ACCESS: Free parking; open sunrise–sunset

MAPS: Posted at trailhead

FACILITIES: Restrooms

WHEELCHAIR ACCESS: None

COMMENTS: Be sure to bring plenty of water on this strenuous, shadeless desert hike, and time it so you are heading back to your car well before dark.

CONTACTS: Bureau of Land Management, Palm Springs, 760-833-7100

Bear Creek Canyon Oasis, La Quinta

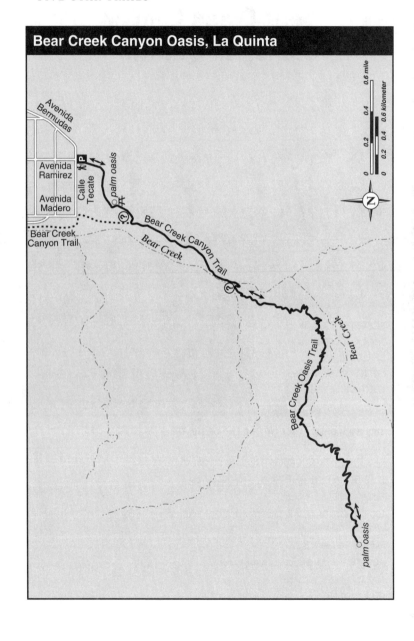

Overview

This popular hike follows a canyon wash, then switchbacks up a series of hillsides, giving way to expansive views of the city of La Quinta and the entire Coachella Valley. While you're likely to see lots of hikers on the Bear Creek Canyon Trail, the turnoff for the Bear Creek Oasis Trail is difficult to spot, so keep your eyes alert for the sign and don't be afraid to ask other hikers if you think you've gone too far and missed it.

Route Details

Begin this hike by following the flat Bear Creek Canyon Trail south toward a cluster of picnic tables and palm oasis on the left (east). After about a quarter-mile, the trail veers to the right, then drops into a wide wash.

Continue south along the west side of the wash (if you stay on the east side, it's easy to miss the turnoff for the oasis). You'll pass several signposts with arrows steering you south to the Bear Creek Oasis Trail. Continue past a rock with faded white paint on it to the right. The trailhead is just past this, after a small cave with more graffiti. A sign and some large rocks mark the start of the trail, which immediately starts ascending the hillside heading southwest. My husband and I missed the turnoff the first time we did this hike,

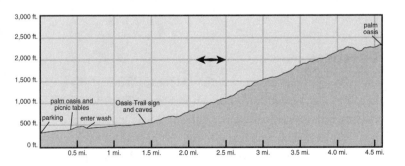

but we turned around and came back to it after seeing other hikers heading down the Oasis path and realizing they would be behind us when they came off the trail.

Once you're on the Bear Creek Oasis Trail, you just want to stay on the trail as it winds up and over the hillsides. This is the strenuous part of the hike, and there will be times (when you're not soaking up the stellar views) when you'll wonder if you're ever going to make it to the oasis. Every turn seems to yield more switchbacks and turns with no end in sight. Some hikers have spotted bighorn sheep here.

After about 3.7 miles, you'll reach 2,000 feet elevation and the oasis will appear in the distance. The trail then dips down across a small wash and heads over a ridge to your final destination: a cool cluster of palm trees alive with birds and plants. From here, retrace your steps back to the parking lot, making sure to allow plenty of time to get back before dark.

Nearby Attractions

Reward yourself after this strenuous desert hike with an ice-cold date shake from **Shields Date Garden** (80-225 S. CA 111; 760-347-7768, **shieldsdategarden.com**). The iconic tourist attraction is a 6-mile drive from the Bear Creek trailhead, on Highway 111 in Indio. Its store sells all kinds of fresh local dates, as well as other seasonal fruits and souvenirs. Sampling is encouraged. An attractive patio café is open for breakfast and lunch.

Directions

From Palm Springs, drive east on CA 111 for 13.75 miles to La Quinta and turn right (south) at Washington Street. Continue about 1.3 miles to Eisenhower Drive, turn right, and drive about 3.6 miles until it ends at Avenida Bermudas. Turn right—the road name changes to Calle Tecate—and after about 0.6 mile, look for the small parking lot to the south. Park here or on the street if the lot is full.

Big Morongo Canyon Trail, Morongo Valley

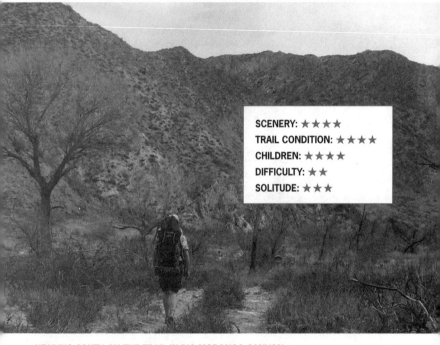

SCENERY: ★ ★ ★
TRAIL CONDITION: ★ ★ ★
CHILDREN: ★ ★ ★
DIFFICULTY: ★ ★
SOLITUDE: ★ ★ ★

HEADING SOUTH ON THE TRAIL IN BIG MORONGO CANYON   Photo: Laura Randall

GPS TRAILHEAD COORDINATES: N34° 03.034' W116° 34.163'

DISTANCE & CONFIGURATION: 2- to 9-mile balloon

HIKING TIME: 2–4 hours

HIGHLIGHTS: Ancient rocks, unique desert wetland, bighorn sheep, 240 species of birds

ELEVATION GAIN: Up to 1,000'

ACCESS: Gates open daily, 7:30 a.m.–sunset

MAPS: Available at kiosk near preserve entrance

FACILITIES: Free parking in lot; restrooms and picnic areas at the entrance

WHEELCHAIR ACCESS: A wheelchair-accessible boardwalk near the entrance runs through the marsh and riparian habitats.

COMMENTS: No pets are allowed. At an elevation of 2,500 feet, the area tends to be 10–20 degrees cooler than Palm Springs and other desert cities.

CONTACTS: Big Morongo Canyon Preserve, 760-363-7190, **bigmorongo.org**

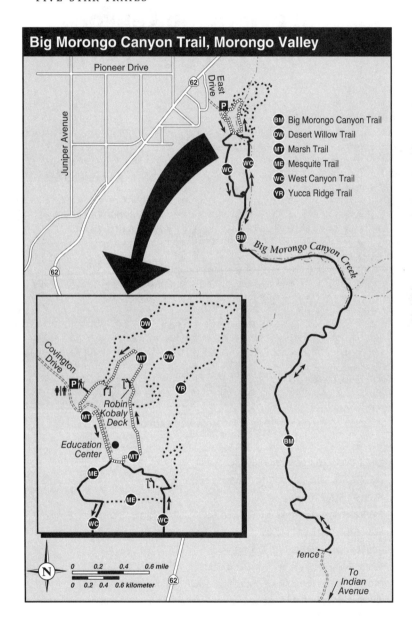

Big Morongo Canyon Trail, Morongo Valley

Pioneer Drive

62

East Drive

Juniper Avenue

BM Big Morongo Canyon Trail
DW Desert Willow Trail
MT Marsh Trail
ME Mesquite Trail
WC West Canyon Trail
YR Yucca Ridge Trail

Big Morongo Canyon Creek

62

Covington Drive

P

Robin Kobaly Deck

Education Center

N

0   0.2   0.4   0.6 mile

0   0.2   0.4   0.6 kilometer

62

fence

To Indian Avenue

Overview

This moderate balloon hike is a good introduction to Big Morongo Preserve, a 29,000-acre desert oasis of marshes, ridges, canyons, and one of the largest cottonwood and willow riparian habitats in California. The preserve is managed by the Bureau of Land Management and helped by a strong corps of volunteers known as Friends of Big Morongo. The hike begins in a quiet marsh, then heads uphill briefly to a saddle ridge before dipping into Big Morongo Canyon and following a stream, fed by snowmelt from the surrounding mountains, 4 miles to Indian Avenue in Desert Hot Springs.

This used to be a popular shuttle hike, but a fence on private property now blocks access to Indian Avenue, and you must turn around at the fence and retrace your route to the parking lot. If you do this hike in the winter or following periods of heavy rain, expect to make several stream crossings and do some slippery rock-scrambling.

OPTION An easy 2- or 3-mile hike can be pieced together on the network of well-marked trails that begins at the entrance kiosk.

Route Details

Grab a trail guide from the kiosk at the preserve entrance and head south on the easy Marsh Trail (actually a boardwalk made of recycled materials). Continue south on the Mesquite Trail from where the

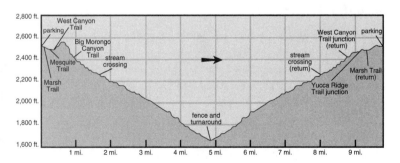

Marsh Trail loops back around to the parking lot, then pick up the West Canyon Trail at about 0.4 mile. Take the sandy trail to the right up the hillside. At about 1 mile from the parking lot, the West Canyon Trail ends and meets up with the main Canyon Trail. Follow it to the right (south) as it descends gradually into the canyon, flanked on either side by fields of creosote bush, willow, alder, and mesquite. You may hear the canyon stream gushing to your left, though the water isn't always visible from the trail. After about 1 mile of meandering south across a wide-open field, the trail crosses the stream and heads due east for about 0.4 mile, then heads south again for the remaining 3 miles. The trail occasionally disappears into brush or sand, but well-placed signposts help prevent serious straying. After passing the 2-mile marker (from the beginning of the Canyon Trail), the trail turns west briefly and hugs the hillside before swerving south again and providing excellent views of the San Jacinto Mountains (snow-capped in winter). From here it's another 2.5 miles of gradual downhill hiking to a fence that blocks access to Indian Avenue. Retrace your route to the main canyon trail, but instead of turning left on the West Canyon Trail, head straight toward the wood fence and follow the Mesquite Trail north. This trail winds past a small nature center and several bird-observation decks with benches. From here it's another 0.6 mile back to the parking lot.

Nearby Attractions

There is an education center and butterfly garden along the Marsh Trail. Docents lead regular bird walks and nature hikes for all levels of hikers; check **bigmorongo.org** for days and times.

Directions

From north Palm Springs, head west on I-10 about 3 miles and take Exit 117 for CA 62/Twentynine Palms. Drive north about 10.5 miles to Morongo Valley and turn right on East Drive. The entrance to the preserve is on the left.

Canyon View Trail, Whitewater Preserve

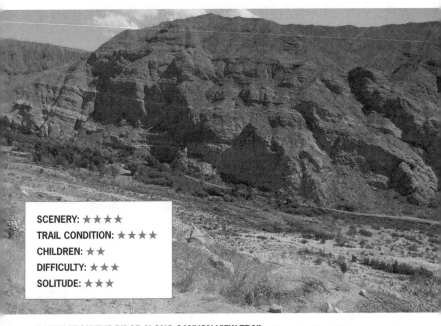

SCENERY: ★ ★ ★ ★
TRAIL CONDITION: ★ ★ ★ ★
CHILDREN: ★ ★
DIFFICULTY: ★ ★ ★
SOLITUDE: ★ ★ ★

A VIEW FROM THE RIDGE ALONG CANYON VIEW TRAIL   Photo: Laura Randall

GPS TRAILHEAD COORDINATES: N33° 59.351' W116° 39.368'

DISTANCE & CONFIGURATION: 3.5-mile loop

HIKING TIME: 2 hours

HIGHLIGHTS: Valley and mountain views, seasonal wildflowers, year-round stream

ELEVATION GAIN: 500'

ACCESS: The preserve is open 8 a.m.–5 p.m. daily, except on major holidays and in the event of dangerous weather conditions. Gates close at 5 p.m. sharp, so time your visit accordingly.

MAPS: At visitor center and trailhead

FACILITIES: Restrooms, picnic area, visitor center with water

WHEELCHAIR ACCESS: Yes, for the first mile

COMMENTS: Make this a kid-friendly 2-mile out-and-back hike by taking it to the first sign for the Pacific Crest Trail and turning around before it gains elevation. This first stretch is completely flat and crisscrosses a stream several times.

CONTACTS: Whitewater Preserve, 760-325-7222, **wildlandsconservancy.org**

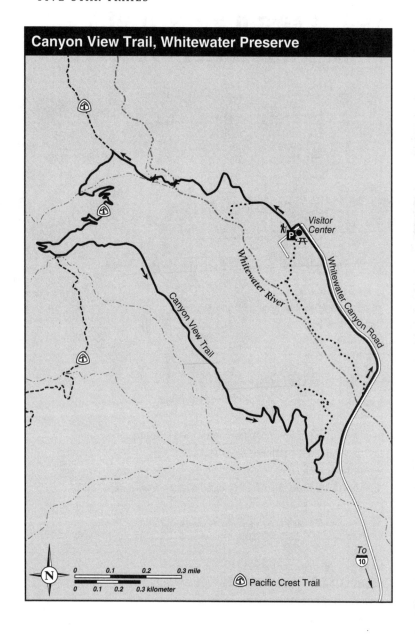

Canyon View Trail, Whitewater Preserve

Visitor Center

Whitewater River

Whitewater Canyon Road

Canyon View Trail

To 10

N

| 0 | 0.1 | 0.2 | 0.3 mile |
| 0 | 0.1 | 0.2 | 0.3 kilometer |

Pacific Crest Trail

Overview

The moderate, well-marked Canyon View Trail is a great introduction to the area and provides a striking contrast to the desert environment of nearby Palm Springs. After a mile of flat trail that crisscrosses a year-round river, it connects with the Pacific Crest Trail (PCT) briefly as it heads south toward Mexico, then loops back along a ridge with spectacular views of the valley. There's a brief stretch at the end that requires walking on the side of the road.

Route Details

Whitewater Preserve is 2,851 acres surrounded by the San Gorgonio Wilderness with the year-round Whitewater River running through it. Park your car in the lot and head to the visitor center to sign the trail register and pick up a map of the area. There's usually water on hand for hikers here. Then head north across the parking lot to the Canyon View Trail. A stone marker etched with a quote from John Muir marks the beginning of this trail, and another boulder reminds you that you're near the PCT, with inscriptions noting that it's 219.1 miles to Mexico and 2,445.4 miles to Canada via the PCT.

The first 0.5 mile of the soft sand-and-rock trail is wide, flat, and attractively lined with white boulders. Follow the signs toward the PCT, and soon you'll come to a wooden footbridge that crosses

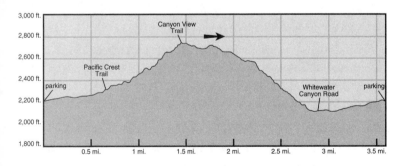

the river. When I hiked this in late spring of a drought year, the river was flowing but easy to cross without getting wet. Continue on the path and you'll come to a junction with the PCT at about two-thirds of a mile from the trailhead. If you've got small children, you might want to turn around here, as the trail now begins its steep 500-foot climb up to the ridge. The trail to the right heads north, eventually reaching the Canadian border. To reach the ridge and intersection with Canyon View Trail, you'll want to head left (south) on the PCT and follow a string of steep switchbacks up to a ridge. (This is the steepest part of the hike.) Once you're at the top, it's smooth sailing (unless you're in the mood for the 200-mile hike down to Mexico). Turn left on the Canyon View Trail—not right on the PCT—and follow it along the ridge accompanied by sweeping mountain and valley views. Keep an eye out for endangered birds like the Southwest willow flycatcher, as well as bighorn sheep, deer, and bear, which roam the corridor between the San Bernardino and San Jacinto Mountains.

After about 0.75 mile of gradual descent, you'll come to Whitewater Canyon Road, the same one you drove on to get to the preserve. It's about a half-mile walk back to the preserve from here.

Nearby Activities

Whitewater Preserve has an attractive picnic area with a trout pond and lots of shade trees. There are no food options around, so pack a lunch and hang out a bit after your hike. If it's early spring, you may run into PCT thru-hikers. **Mission Creek Preserve,** also run by the Wildlands Conservancy, is just a few miles to the northeast, and both properties link to the PCT.

Directions

The preserve is about 16 miles northwest of Palm Springs. Get on I-10 West and take Exit 114 toward Whitewater. Turn right on Tipton Road, then make a left onto Whitewater Canyon Road and follow it north 4.5 miles until it ends at the preserve.

16

Desert Hot Springs Loop, Desert Hot Springs

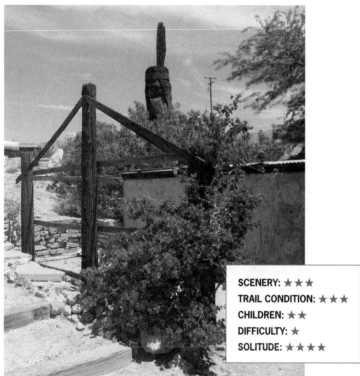

SCENERY: ★★★
TRAIL CONDITION: ★★★
CHILDREN: ★★
DIFFICULTY: ★
SOLITUDE: ★★★★

CABOT'S PUEBLO MUSEUM SITS NEAR A NETWORK OF TRAILS.

GPS TRAILHEAD COORDINATES: N33° 58.357' W116° 29.515'
DISTANCE & CONFIGURATION: 1.2-mile loop
HIKING TIME: 45 minutes–1 hour
HIGHLIGHTS: Views of Palm Springs and surrounding mountains, desert vegetation, solitude
ELEVATION GAIN: 200'
ACCESS: 24/7, dogs allowed
MAPS: None
FACILITIES: None
WHEELCHAIR ACCESS: None
CONTACTS: Desert Hot Springs Chamber of Commerce, 760-329-6403

Desert Hot Springs Loop, Desert Hot Springs

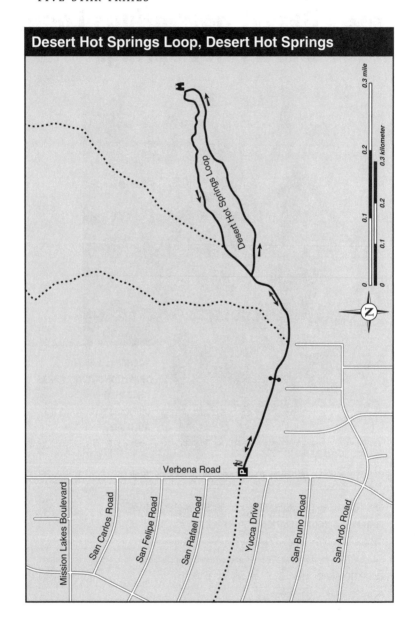

Desert Hot Springs Loop

Verbena Road

Mission Lakes Boulevard

San Carlos Road

San Felipe Road

San Rafael Road

Yucca Drive

San Bruno Road

San Ardo Road

0.3 mile
0.1   0.2
0.3 kilometer
0   0.1   0.2

Overview

This easy balloon hike begins on the northeast edge of town and follows a flat trail past desert scrub to a small hill that overlooks Palm Springs and the San Jacinto Mountains. Bring a companion (human or canine) and plenty of water on this shadeless, often-deserted hike.

Route Details

A small, rapidly developing town north of Palm Springs, Desert Hot Springs has a couple of decent hiking trails that afford unique views of Palm Springs and its surrounding mountains and windmill farms. Karl and Ursula Furrer of the now-closed Swiss Health Resort first introduced me to the hiking trails in Desert Hot Springs on an early December morning, when the air was chilly and clear. It had snowed in the surrounding mountains the night before, and we were treated to gorgeous views of white-capped peaks to the south and northwest. The couple had been walking the trails to the north and east of their small hotel for decades with their two dogs and any hotel guest who wanted to join them.

While a coat and hat might be necessary in winter, be mindful that Desert Hot Springs hits the triple digits in summer and early fall. Avoid hiking during these months, or go very early in the morning to avoid the crushing heat.

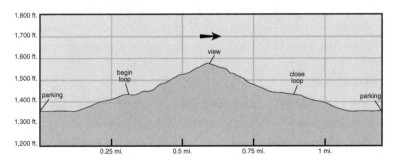

97

Pick up the flat sand-and-rock trail on the east side of Verbena Drive and follow it east toward a series of scrub-covered hills. The trail briefly skirts a chain-link fence, then begins a gradual ascent before bearing left and following a wide dirt road away from the residential development.

At 0.4 mile, turn right from the dirt road onto a narrow trail leading due east. Go straight for about 0.3 mile, then veer right up a short hill graced by a small clearing. You won't likely be tired at this point, but take time to stop and admire the expansive views of Palm Springs and the San Jacinto Mountains. The windmill farms visible from here sit in San Gorgonio Pass, one of the most consistently windy spots in the world.

Follow the trail west from here, and then head south as it descends toward the scrub-covered canyon and loops back to the main dirt road. Turn left at the dirt road and retrace your route past the chain-link fence to the trailhead.

Nearby Attractions

Just around the corner from the trailhead **Cabot's Pueblo Museum** (760-329-7610, **cabotsmuseum.org**) is a quirky destination worth a visit in its own right. It's a Hopi-inspired adobe complex of 35 rooms that visionary homesteader Cabot Yerxa built by hand in 1941, using repurposed materials he found in the desert; Yerxa worked on the project until his death in 1965 at age 81. The exhibits include a large collection of Native American pottery and early-20th-century photographs. Tours are held daily (hours are limited during the summer).

Directions

From I-10, take Palm Drive north about 6.1 miles through Desert Hot Springs. Make a right on Eighth Street and continue about 0.5 mile to Verbena Drive. Turn left on Verbena Drive and go about four blocks. Park on the street. The trailhead begins on the east side of Verbena Drive, just north of Yucca Drive.

Hopalong Cassidy Trail, Palm Desert

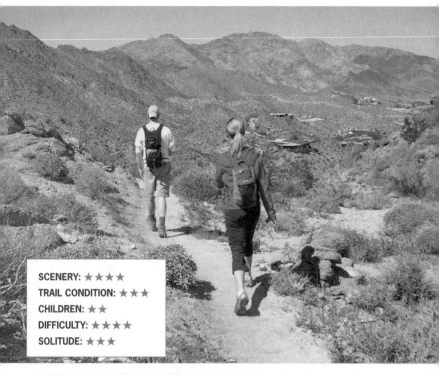

SCENERY: ★ ★ ★ ★
TRAIL CONDITION: ★ ★ ★
CHILDREN: ★ ★
DIFFICULTY: ★ ★ ★ ★
SOLITUDE: ★ ★ ★

VIEWS OF PALM DESERT WEAVE IN AND OUT OF SIGHT ALONG THE HOPALONG CASSIDY TRAIL. Photo: Eric Forsberg

GPS TRAILHEAD COORDINATES: N33° 43.530' W116° 24.367'

DISTANCE & CONFIGURATION: 2- to 4-mile out-and-back

HIKING TIME: 1–3 hours

HIGHLIGHTS: Sweeping views of Coachella Valley, desert vegetation, rock formations

ELEVATION GAIN: 400'

ACCESS: Free parking; open sunrise–sunset

MAPS: None

FACILITIES: None

WHEELCHAIR ACCESS: None

CONTACTS: Palm Desert Visitor Center, 760-568-1441 or 800-873-2428, **palm-desert.org;** Bureau of Land Management, 760-862-9984

Hopalong Cassidy Trail, Palm Desert

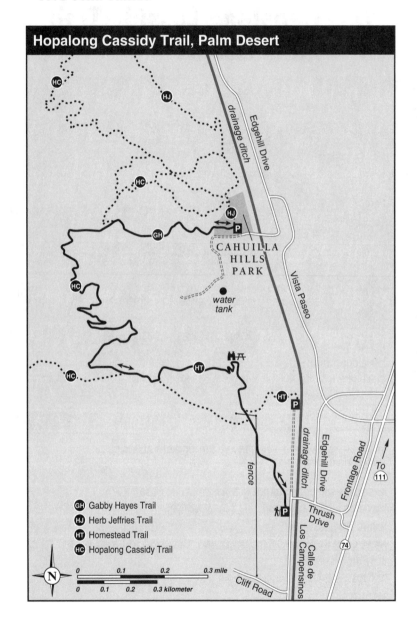

CAHUILLA
HILLS
PARK

water
tank

Edgehill Drive

drainage ditch

Vista Paseo

fence

drainage ditch

Edgehill Drive

Frontage Road

To
111

Thrush
Drive

Calle de
Los Campensinos

Cliff Road

74

GH Gabby Hayes Trail
HJ Herb Jeffries Trail
HT Homestead Trail
HC Hopalong Cassidy Trail

N

| 0 | 0.1 | 0.2 | 0.3 mile |
| 0 | 0.1 | 0.2 | 0.3 kilometer |

Overview

This short but strenuous hike begins on the Art Smith Trail at the base of an off-leash dog park in Palm Desert and links with the 8-mile Hopalong Cassidy Trail, which opened in 2006 as a connector to the Art Smith and Mirage Trails.

Route Details

Look for the large ART SMITH TRAIL sign at the northern end of the park and follow the sand trail north as it parallels a wooden fence. Soon you'll come to a gap in the fence; go through it and then follow the narrow trail up a steep hill covered in rocks and desert vegetation. At 0.25 mile, the narrow trail ends at a gated fire road. Walk around the gate and continue up the fire road to a scenic overlook with a picnic table, thatched roof overhang, and spectacular views of Palm Desert and the sprawling Coachella Valley. From here the trail narrows and continues to switchback up the hillside to the west. At 0.4 mile, the path levels briefly, then begins to climb again. You'll see a large water tank below you to the right.

At about 0.7 mile, the trail splits, with the left branch continuing uphill to connect with the Trail to the Cross (on which dogs are prohibited). This trail provides stellar views of the valley and San

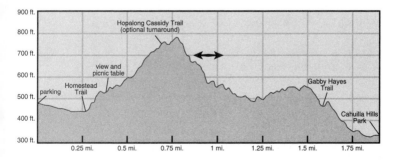

Jacinto Mountains to the west, but it is a steep quarter-mile climb to nowhere—it ends abruptly at a chain-link fence bordering a nearby golf course.

Hikers with dogs will want to turn back at the split or bear right on the Hopalong Cassidy Trail, which travels down the canyon and links with the Gabby Hayes Trail. The Gabby Hayes Trail leads down to Cahuilla Hills Park, at 45-825 Edgehill Dr. in Palm Desert. From here you can retrace your route to Homme-Adams Park (for a total of 4 miles), or arrange to be picked up at Cahuilla Hills Park.

Directions

From I-10, take Exit 131/Monterey Avenue in Palm Desert and drive south about 5.9 miles. After crossing Palm Canyon Drive (CA 111), continue south about 1.1 mile, now on Pines to Palms Highway (CA 74), to Thrush Road. Turn right, then stay on Thrush as it jogs to the right, then turns left toward the mountains. Follow the road across a small bridge to Homme-Adams Park, then turn left and park in the small lot on the right side of the road.

18

Mirage Trail (Bump and Grind), Palm Desert

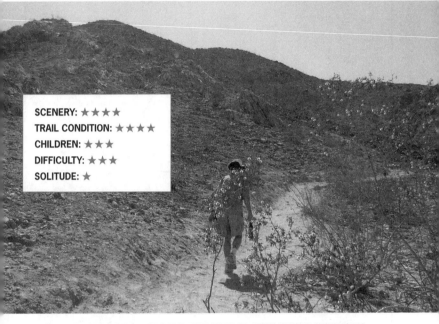

EARLY ELEVATION GAIN ALONG THE MIRAGE TRAIL GIVES WAY TO PANORAMIC VALLEY VIEWS. Photo: Laura Randall

SCENERY: ★ ★ ★ ★
TRAIL CONDITION: ★ ★ ★ ★
CHILDREN: ★ ★ ★
DIFFICULTY: ★ ★ ★
SOLITUDE: ★

GPS TRAILHEAD COORDINATES: N33° 43.530' W116° 24.367'

DISTANCE & CONFIGURATION: 3-mile loop

HIKING TIME: 1 hour

HIGHLIGHTS: Expansive views of the desert and mountains, desert vegetation, spring wildflowers

ELEVATION GAIN: 900'

ACCESS: Trailhead open sunrise–sunset

MAPS: At trailhead kiosk

FACILITIES: Free street parking on Painter's Path behind the Desert Crossing Shopping Center; no restrooms or water

WHEELCHAIR ACCESS: None

COMMENTS: No dogs or other pets are allowed on the trail. The trail surrounds a bighorn sheep habitat; Fish & Wildlife officials installed a gate near the upper trail to block access.

CONTACTS: Palm Desert Visitor Center, 760-568-1441 or 800-873-2428, **palm-desert.org**

Mirage Trail Loop (Bump and Grind), Palm Desert

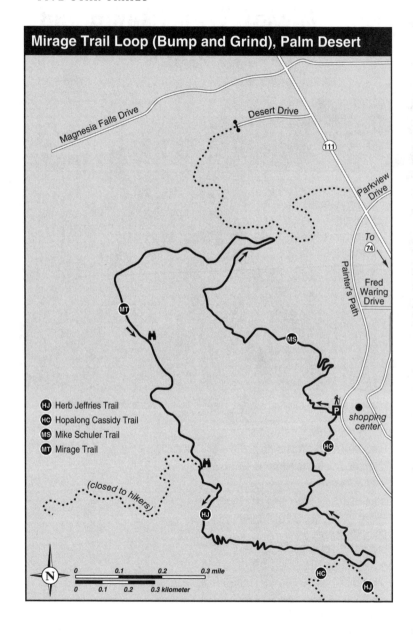

HJ Herb Jeffries Trail
HC Hopalong Cassidy Trail
MS Mike Schuler Trail
MT Mirage Trail

(closed to hikers)

Magnesia Falls Drive

Desert Drive

111

Parkview Drive

To 74

Painter's Path

Fred Waring Drive

shopping center

P

N

| 0 | 0.1 | 0.2 | 0.3 mile |
| 0 | 0.1 | 0.2 | 0.3 kilometer |

Overview

This popular local hike features a gradual 900-foot ascent via switch-backs to a wide-open clearing with spectacular views of the Coachella Valley and San Jacinto Mountains. It is well maintained and has several lookout points to stop and soak up the scenery along the way. Don't come here for solitude, especially on weekends. It's very popular with locals as a place to get a regular cardio workout.

Route Details

This trail is officially called the Mirage Trail, though locals refer to it as the "Bump and Grind." It used to be accessible via a residential area in Rancho Mirage on Magnesia Falls Drive, but that trailhead closed; therefore, the easiest way to access it now is from Painter's Path in Palm Desert, behind the Desert Crossing Shopping Center.

After parking, look for the large stone monument and map near the trailhead.

Follow the Mike Schuler Trail to the right as it winds up the hill-side. (The Hopalong Cassidy Trail heads left and loops back around in clockwise fashion, but it's a steeper climb up the hill.) The trail is wide and well-maintained and soon yields terrific wide-open views of the valley and mountains.

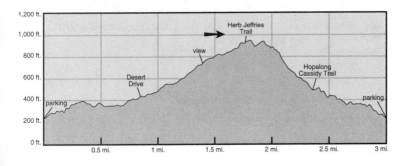

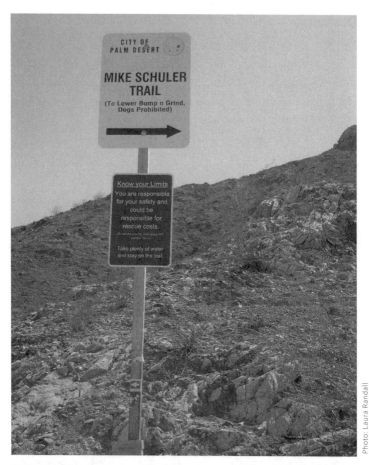

Photo: Laura Randall

MOST MIRAGE TRAIL HIKERS OPT TO TAKE THE COUNTERCLOCKWISE ROUTE THAT BEGINS AT MIKE SCHULER TRAIL.

After you cross the wash, you'll immediately start climbing up the rocky hillside via easy switchbacks. After about 0.4 mile, the trail levels and meets up with the wider trail that begins at Desert Drive. Follow the trail left as it winds up the mountain. Soon you'll come to a wide clearing on the left with views of the Coachella Valley. There's no need to stop here unless you want to, as there are more (and better) viewpoints about every quarter-mile. As you continue up the mountain, you'll notice narrower paths that branch off here and there from the main trail. Most of them eventually just loop back to the main trail. At 0.7 mile, you'll reach another clearing with good views; from here the trail continues to weave uphill along the mountain ridge. For the next half-mile or so, views of the Coachella Valley to the north accompany you as the trail makes a series of long switchbacks. The San Jacinto Mountains weave in and out of sight to the west. Soon you reach another lookout, this one with a view east toward the Salton Sea. Just past this lookout, a trail forks left and heads east over a hillside.

Continue west on the Bump and Grind Trail, past another viewpoint that overlooks the lower part of the route. At about 1.2 miles, the trail comes to another viewpoint, this one facing northeast. Look to the east for good views of the golf courses and palm-lined hotel complexes that make up the resort town of La Quinta. As you near the top, you'll see a fence with a small sign that reads ECOLOGICAL RESERVE. Continue on the main trail to a small clearing. Soak up the views once more before picking up the Hopalong Cassidy Trail for the steep descent back to civilization.

Nearby Attractions

This trailhead is surrounded by commercial shopping and eating options. **The River at Rancho Mirage,** just across Highway 111, is a sprawling complex of restaurants, shops, and a movie theater. Also nearby, the **Palm Desert Visitor Center** (73-470 El Paseo) has good hiking maps of the area and is a reliable source for updates on trail conditions and reroutes; it's open 10 a.m.–6 p.m. Monday–Saturday.

Directions

From I-10, take Exit 131/Monterey Avenue and drive south about 5.3 miles. Make a right on Fred Waring Drive and follow it about 0.8 mile west to Painter's Path. Make a left and drive about 0.5 mile until you see the trailhead on the right. Park on the street.

19

Randall Henderson Loop, Palm Desert

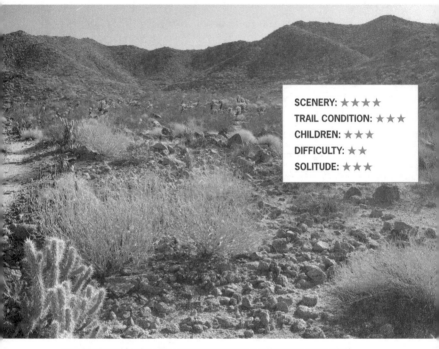

SCENERY: ★★★★
TRAIL CONDITION: ★★★
CHILDREN: ★★★
DIFFICULTY: ★★
SOLITUDE: ★★★

DESERT VEGETATION AND MOUNTAIN VIEWS FROM THE MODERATE RANDALL HENDERSON TRAIL Photo: Barbi Lynn Lazarus

GPS TRAILHEAD COORDINATES: N33° 40.291' W116° 24.474'

DISTANCE & CONFIGURATION: 3-mile loop

HIKING TIME: 1–2 hours

HIGHLIGHTS: Ocotillo trees, cacti, and other desert vegetation, plus mountain views and a habitat for endangered Peninsular bighorn sheep

ELEVATION GAIN: 400'

ACCESS: Trailhead open sunrise–sunset

MAPS: Available at visitor center

FACILITIES: Visitor center with restrooms and parking lot

WHEELCHAIR ACCESS: None

COMMENTS: Hats and sunscreen are a must for this shadeless hike.

CONTACTS: Santa Rosa and San Jacinto Mountains National Monument, 760-862-9984

Randall Henderson Loop, Palm Desert

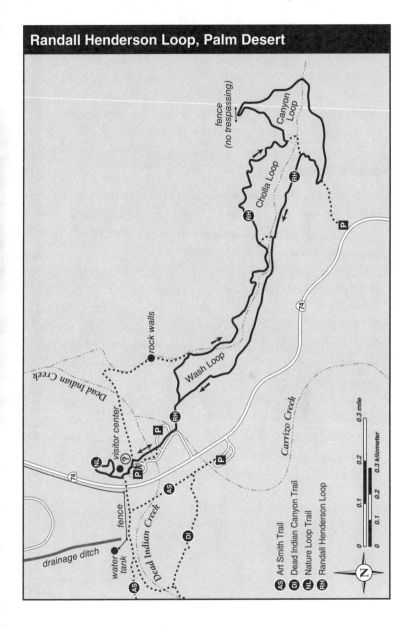

fence
(no trespassing)

Canyon Loop

Cholla Loop

RH

RH

P

74

rock walls

Dead Indian Creek

Wash Loop

Carrizo Creek

visitor center

RH

P

NL

P

74

P

fence

AS

Dead Indian Creek

DI

drainage ditch

water tank

AS

AS Art Smith Trail
DI Dead Indian Canyon Trail
NL Nature Loop Trail
RH Randall Henderson Loop

0   0.1   0.2   0.3 mile
0   0.1   0.2   0.3 kilometer

N

Overview

This loop hike near a visitor center is a good introduction to desert hiking, with a variety of plants and flowers, an easy-to-follow trail, and a moderate elevation gain of 400 feet. It skirts a major habitat for endangered Peninsular bighorn sheep: Heed the warnings and stay on the marked trail. Dogs aren't allowed on the trail.

Route Details

Begin this hike by walking the short quarter-mile nature loop trail behind the visitor center. Signs identify many of the desert plants and flowers you will see on the trail, such as sandpaper plants, brittle bush, creosote bush, and many varieties of cacti.

Proceed to the Randall Henderson Trailhead, on the eastern side of the parking lot in front of the visitor center. Look for the large kiosk with maps of Palm Desert and descriptions of the area's plants and wildlife. Follow the soft, sandy trail southeast as it skirts the parking lot. (You can also pick up the trail along the driveway leading to the visitor center, closer to CA 74.) Soon you will come to a fork—opt for the left trail, which begins to climb moderately along a wash to a narrow canyon. This part of the trail might require some moderate rock scrambling. You can also see CA 74 from here, but it's far enough away to be unintrusive. After another half-mile or so, you'll come to another trail junction that links up with the right trail from the first fork. Stay to the left; the path to the right takes you back to the parking lot.

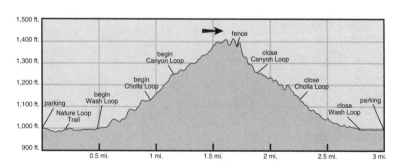

After another brief climb, the trail levels and follows a saddle ridge for about 0.3 mile, then heads north up wide switchbacks to the trail's high point. Teddy-bear cholla cactus are scattered throughout this area. Also known as jumping cholla, they are called "teddy bear" because their spiny stems appear soft from a distance. You'll also see lots of chuparosa shrubs, creosote bush, and sandpaper plants along this part of the trail.

The trip back down the mountain begins when you reach a sign and a fence blocking public access. Continue on the trail as it loops back down the mountain. Look for the green spiny branches of ocotillo trees, which spike with red flowers in the spring, on either side of the path.

At about 1.8 miles from the trailhead, you'll come to a trail junction. Stay right and continue another quarter-mile downhill to the desert floor. At this point the route crosses a few large boulders; it's easiest to scoot down them on your behind, especially if you're not wearing hiking boots. From here the trail reconnects with the trail you followed on the way in, and it's another 1.2 miles of flat hiking back to the visitor center.

Nearby Attractions

The **National Monument Visitor Center** (51500 CA 74) offers information about hiking in the Palm Springs–Desert Cities area. Rangers are on hand to answer questions and lead fun activities like scorpion hunts and nighttime nature hikes. A gift shop sells books, maps, and promotional materials, and an easy walking path studded with native plants is in the back. Visit **www.desertmountains.org** for more information.

Directions

From I-10, take Exit 131/Monterey Avenue in Palm Desert and drive south about 5.9 miles. After crossing Palm Canyon Drive (CA 111), continue south as the road becomes Pines to Palms Highway (CA 74) and drive another 3.5 miles to the visitor center for the Santa Rosa and San Jacinto Mountains National Monument. Turn left and follow the long driveway to the parking lot.

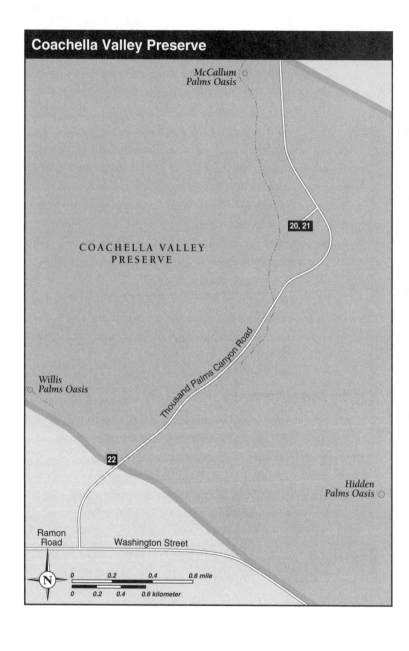

Coachella Valley Preserve

McCallum
Palms Oasis

20, 21

COACHELLA VALLEY
PRESERVE

Thousand Palms Canyon Road

Willis
Palms Oasis

22

Hidden
Palms Oasis

Ramon
Road

Washington Street

N

| 0 | 0.2 | 0.4 | 0.6 mile |
| 0 | 0.2 | 0.4 | 0.6 kilometer |

Coachella Valley Preserve

MOST TRAILS IN COACHELLA VALLEY PRESERVE LEAD TO THICK PALM OASES.

Photo: Laura Randall

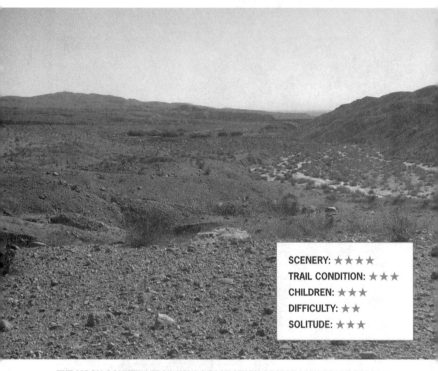

SCENERY: ★ ★ ★ ★
TRAIL CONDITION: ★ ★ ★
CHILDREN: ★ ★ ★
DIFFICULTY: ★ ★
SOLITUDE: ★ ★ ★

THE MOON COUNTRY TRAIL WINDS PAST STARK DESERT LANDSCAPE BEFORE ENDING AT A SHADY GROVE OF DESERT FAN PALMS. Photo: Laura Randall

GPS TRAILHEAD COORDINATES: N33° 50.252' W116° 18.514'

DISTANCE & CONFIGURATION: 2- to 4.2-mile balloon

HIKING TIME: 45 minutes–2 hours

HIGHLIGHTS: Desert fan palms, sandy wash, sand dunes, pond

ELEVATION GAIN: 300'

ACCESS: The visitor center and gates are closed June–August, but hikers can still access the preserve and trails by parking on Ramon Road. Admission is free.

MAPS: At visitor center or **coachellavalleypreserve.org**

FACILITIES: Parking lot, restrooms, and water

WHEELCHAIR ACCESS: None

COMMENTS: An easier kid-friendly alternative to the Moon Country Trail is the 2-mile round-trip McCallum Trail, which leads directly to the palm oasis, then returns to the visitor center.

CONTACTS: Coachella Valley Preserve, 760-343-2733, **coachellavalleypreserve.org**

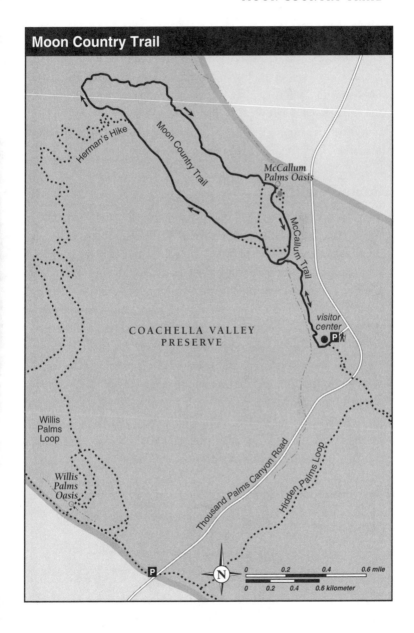

Moon Country Trail

Herman's Hike

Moon Country Trail

McCallum
Palms Oasis

McCallum Trail

visitor
center

COACHELLA VALLEY
PRESERVE

Willis
Palms
Loop

Willis
Palms
Oasis

Hidden Palms Loop

Thousand Palms Canyon Road

N

| 0 | 0.2 | 0.4 | 0.6 mile |

| 0 | 0.2 | 0.4 | 0.6 kilometer |

Overview

This mostly flat trail crosses the San Andreas Fault and loops around a sandy wash before leading to one of the largest groves of desert fan palms in California and a picture-perfect pond that is home to the endangered desert pupfish. The trail can be shortened to 2 miles round-trip by skipping the Moon Country segment and following the McCallum Trail straight to the palm grove.

Route Details

The Moon Country Trail is one of several well-maintained trails within the Coachella Valley Preserve, a 20,000-acre property made up of sand dunes, groves of desert fan palms, and an array of wildlife that includes the rare fringe-toed lizard. Begin your hike under the grove of palm trees off the main parking lot, where you'll find a staffed nature center (open most days), maps, and restrooms. To get to the Moon Country Trail, take the McCallum Trail to the right of the nature center. The sandy trail begins in the shade of palm trees that are believed to be 250 years old. After crossing a couple of wooden bridges, you will come to a fork: Follow the McCallum Trail straight (north).

At 0.3 mile, the trail leaves the shade and widens as it climbs a small hill to a junction. The trail to the right leads back to the parking lot. You want to continue straight.

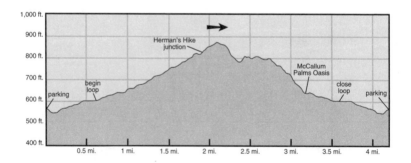

Low-lying smoke trees (known for their ash-colored stems) and creosote bushes line the trail. Also here are cattle spinach, a desert weed that sprouts yellow flowers from May to October, and arrow weed. At about 0.5 mile, you'll pass a private home on the right. Continue straight past the driveway, then follow the trail to the left and up a small hill. After another few hundred feet, you will come to another junction. The McCallum Palms Oasis is straight ahead. To get to the Moon Country Trail, take the left fork and go up another small hill. You'll see a small sign for the Moon Country Trail; stay left and follow the canyon wash west. The sandy trail becomes a wide canyon wash that is bordered by brown hillsides and desert scrub. You may think you've wandered off the main trail at times; just keep heading straight (west) and you'll be fine. Look closely at the landscape and you'll see how floods passed through this area at some point: The ground is cracked and many of the bushes lean toward the east. After 2 miles, you'll see a signpost on the right; walk past it and continue north up a narrow, rock-lined trail that winds up a short hillside. From here the trail heads back to the east, and you can see the McCallum Palms Oasis in the distance as you head back down the north side of the hill. Now the Little San Bernardino Mountains and Coachella Valley are in full view, as are the flat-top rock formations that dot the landscape north of Thousand Palms Canyon Road. At 2.8 miles, you'll reach a lookout point; from here the trail heads downhill and becomes sandy.

At 3 miles, the trail levels and passes the sand dunes that are a critical habitat for the fringe-toed lizard. Anyone caught trespassing on the dunes will be fined. Follow the trail left as it enters McCallum Palms Oasis. Among the first things you will see as you enter the grove are piles of dry palm fronds; they provide shelter and nesting materials for some of the animals who live in the preserve. Soon the path winds past a pond on the left. This is good place to stop and look for tadpoles and the endangered desert pupfish, a minnowlike fish whose population is dwindling. The trail continues to meander in the shade for another 0.3 mile before reconnecting with the trail that will return you to the parking lot.

Nearby Attractions

Before heading out, take the time to visit the **Palm House Visitor Center** if it's open. Housed in a 1930s log cabin, it has maps, wildlife displays, and a working icebox that is about as old as the cabin.

Directions

From I-10, take Exit 130/Ramon Road and head east on Ramon about 4.3 miles to Thousand Palms Canyon Road. Turn left and continue to the preserve's main entrance.

Pushawalla Palms Loop

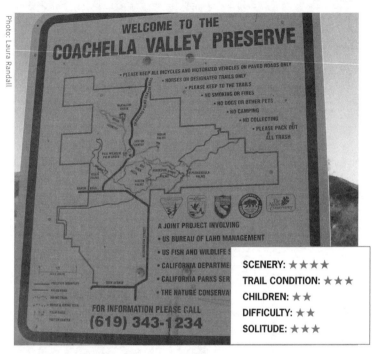

SCENERY: ★ ★ ★ ★
TRAIL CONDITION: ★ ★ ★
CHILDREN: ★ ★
DIFFICULTY: ★ ★
SOLITUDE: ★ ★ ★

MAPS AND WELL-MAINTAINED TRAILS HELP VISITORS NAVIGATE THE 20,000-ACRE PRESERVE.

GPS TRAILHEAD COORDINATES: N33° 50.123' W116° 18.367'

DISTANCE & CONFIGURATION: 6-mile loop

HIKING TIME: 2 hours

HIGHLIGHTS: Palm groves, desert and mountain views, Mission Creek earthquake fault

ELEVATION GAIN: 450'

ACCESS: The visitor center and gates are closed June–August, but hikers can still access the preserve and trails by parking on Ramon Road. Admission is free.

MAPS: At visitor center or **coachellavalleypreserve.org**

FACILITIES: Parking lot, restrooms, and water

WHEELCHAIR ACCESS: None

COMMENTS: Instead of looping north at Pushawalla Palms, follow the signs for Horseshoe Palms to the west, just before the entrance to the Pushawalla Palms grove. This heads southwest past Horseshoe and Hidden Palms, then loops north to rejoin the Pushawalla Trail just before the parking pullout. The round-trip total of this loop hike is 4.3 miles.

CONTACTS: Coachella Valley Preserve, 760-343-2733, **coachellavalleypreserve.org**

Pushawalla Palms Loop

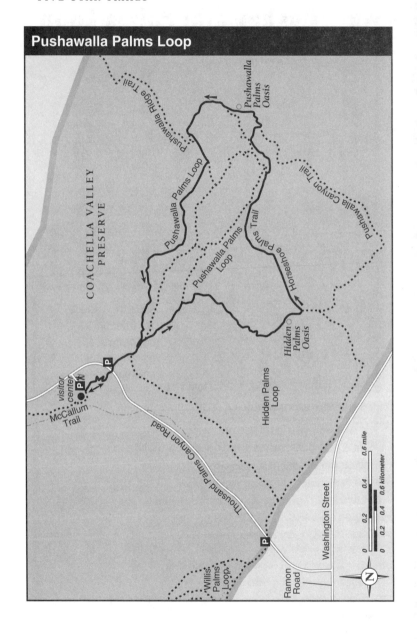

Overview

The Pushawalla Palms Trail is one of several well-maintained trails within the Coachella Valley Preserve, a 20,000-acre property that is home to sand dunes, groves of desert fan palms, and an array of wildlife that includes the rare fringe-toed lizard. It begins near the visitor center and follows the ridge of an uplifted earthquake fault, past stunning views of the Coachella Valley down to a large palm grove, then returns via a scrub-covered wash. I like to do this hike in late afternoon, when the sinking sun casts dramatic shadows over the desert and the San Bernardino Mountains.

Route Details

Pick up a map of the preserve's trail system at the Palm House Visitor Center on Thousand Palms Canyon Road, and look for signs marking the start of the Pushawalla Palms Trail on the southeast side of the parking lot. Cross Thousand Palms Road to the official start of the trail. There is also a parking pullout at the trailhead. Start walking southeast across a wash filled with cacti and brush toward what looks like a low mountain ridge. Follow the signs for the Pushawalla and Horseshoe Palms Trails (a signed trail leading to Hidden Palms branches right soon after you begin). After about 0.5 mile, you will

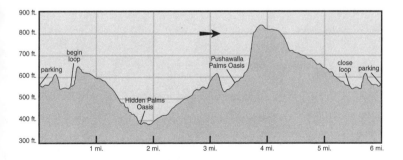

reach a flight of wooden steps that leads straight up the fault ridge. At the top, the trail follows the ridge for about 1 mile, past terrific views of the Coachella Valley to the south and the Little San Bernardino Mountains to the north. You are walking along an uplifted edge of the Mission Creek earthquake fault, a branch of the San Andreas fault system. After about 0.5 mile, the Hidden Palms Oasis is below you on the right. There are no clearings or resting areas along the ridge, but the entire walk is one big photo opportunity—there is no bad angle. Continue walking east another 0.5 mile or so until the trail dips back down to the canyon floor. At the bottom, the trail splits. Head right (southeast) to continue down to Pushawalla Palms Trail, following a dry, rock-filled streambed for about 0.3 mile until it becomes a sandy trail that leads to the palm grove. Follow the trail north from here as it skirts the entire palm grove and loops back to the canyon wash. At the trail split near the fault ridge, take the sandy right-hand path back toward the visitor center. The earthquake fault ridge that you followed on the way in will be on your left. The views are somewhat less interesting on the walk back to the nature center, but you will see a variety of desert vegetation, from cacti to desert lavender to creosote bush. A prominent landmark is a tall scorched palm trunk that stands by itself between the wash trail and the fault ridge. From here it's another mile back to the visitor center.

Nearby Activities

See previous hike.

Directions

From I-10, take Exit 130/Ramon Road and head east on Ramon about 4.3 miles to Thousand Palms Canyon Road. Turn left and continue to the preserve's main entrance.

Willis Palms Loop

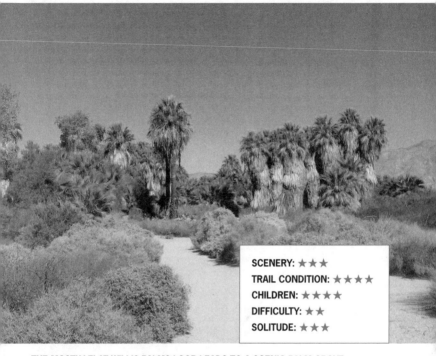

SCENERY: ★ ★ ★
TRAIL CONDITION: ★ ★ ★ ★
CHILDREN: ★ ★ ★ ★
DIFFICULTY: ★ ★
SOLITUDE: ★ ★ ★

THE MOSTLY FLAT WILLIS PALMS LOOP LEADS TO A SCENIC PALM GROVE.
Photo: Laura Randall

GPS TRAILHEAD COORDINATES: N33° 49.330' W116° 19.375'

DISTANCE & CONFIGURATION: 2- to 4.75-mile balloon

HIKING TIME: 1–1.5 hours

HIGHLIGHTS: Palm grove, desert vegetation, mountain views

ELEVATION GAIN: 250'–440'

ACCESS: The visitor center and gates are closed June–August, but hikers can still access the preserve and trails by parking on Ramon Road. Admission is free.

MAPS: At visitor center or **coachellavalleypreserve.org**

FACILITIES: Parking lot, restrooms, and water

WHEELCHAIR ACCESS: None

COMMENTS: This can also be an easy, flat 2-mile hike by turning around at the western edge of the palm grove and retracing your route to the trailhead.

CONTACTS: Coachella Valley Preserve, 760-343-2733, **coachellavalleypreserve.org**

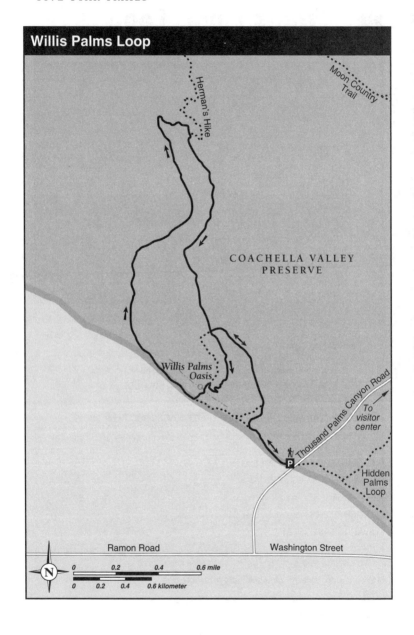

Willis Palms Loop

Herman's Hike

Moon Country Trail

COACHELLA VALLEY
PRESERVE

Willis Palms
Oasis

Thousand Palms Canyon Road

To
visitor
center

P

Hidden
Palms
Loop

Ramon Road

Washington Street

N

| 0 | 0.2 | 0.4 | 0.6 mile |
| 0 | 0.2 | 0.4 | 0.6 kilometer |

Overview

The Willis Palms Loop is an easy hike to a beautiful palm oasis within the Coachella Valley Preserve trail system. The loop requires a moderate scramble up a rocky hillside, but the rest of the route is mostly flat and easy to follow. No dogs are allowed. Traffic noise from Ramon Road and views of electric towers mar the first leg of the hike, but the hike gets more secluded and scenic once it reaches the palm grove.

Route Details

The Coachella Valley Preserve is a 20,000-acre property that is home to sand dunes, groves of desert fan palms, and an array of wildlife that includes the rare fringe-toed lizard. Admission is free. There are several trails within the preserve; Willis Palms is one of the few that doesn't begin in the main parking lot on Thousand Palms Road.

Look for the trailhead just beyond the gate bordering the parking pullout on Thousand Palms Road. Begin walking northwest along a sandy wash toward the palm grove. At 0.25 mile, you'll come to a fork; bear right and up a small hill. At this point, you're heading north, away from the palm grove, but the trail soon curves back to

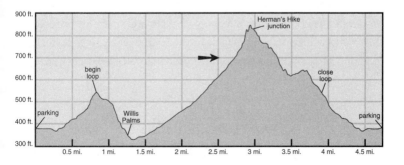

the south. At 0.4 mile, the trail splits again; head left (south) toward Ramon Road and continue 0.2 mile toward the palm oasis. Look for a small signpost to the southwest and follow the trail as it winds along the south side of the palm grove. At 0.9 mile, you'll reach the far western end of the grove, marked by a rusty post and a separate sign alerting you that there's a habitat restoration in progress. From here, you can retrace your route to the parking lot for an easy 2-mile hike or follow the trail uphill to the cool, protected shade of the palm grove. After exploring the grove, continue on the trail as it heads northwest out of the palm grove, then veers to the right (north), gently climbing a rocky hillside. This part of the trail takes you deeper into the preserve and is the most secluded part of the hike. At about 1.8 miles, the trail loops back and heads south toward the palm grove, following the base of a rocky hill. It reconnects with the main trail at 2.7 miles and heads southeast to the parking pullout.

Nearby Attractions

See Hikes 20 and 21 (pages 114 and 119).

Directions

From I-10, take Exit 130/Ramon Road and head east on Ramon about 4.3 miles to Thousand Palms Canyon Road. Turn left and continue about 0.4 mile until you see a small sign for Coachella Valley Preserve. Park in the small pullout on the left (west) side of the road. Maps and restrooms are available at the visitor center, which you'll find on Thousand Palms Canyon Road about 1 mile ahead.

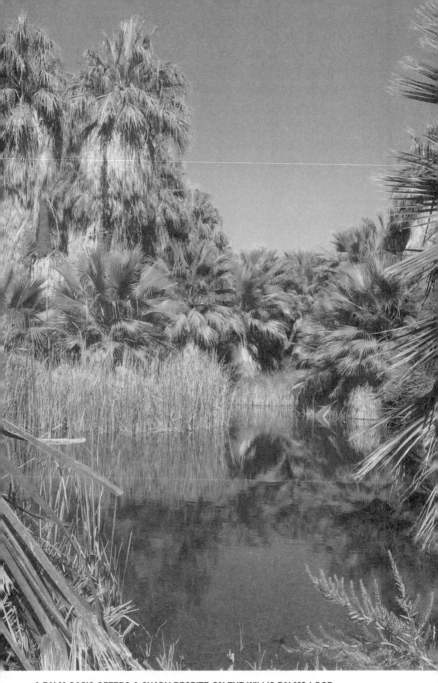

A PALM OASIS OFFERS A SHADY RESPITE ON THE WILLIS PALMS LOOP.

Photo: Laura Randall

Santa Rosa and San Jacinto Mountains

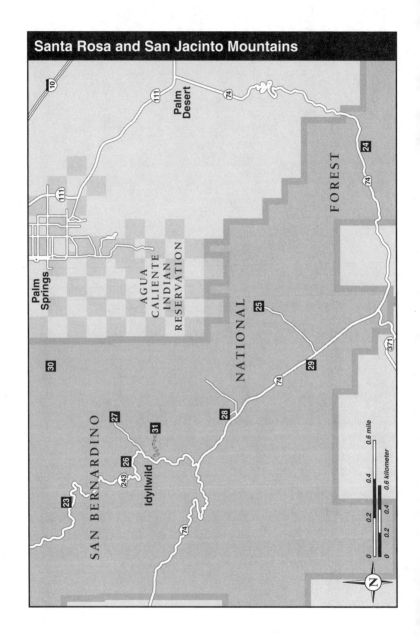

Santa Rosa and
San Jacinto Mountains

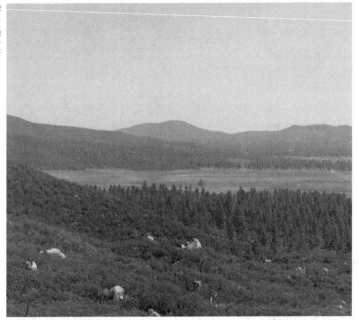

VIEWS OF PINE FOREST AND LAKE HEMET FROM THE HURKEY CREEK TRAIL
(See Hike 28, page 151.)

Photo: Chris Hogan

Black Mountain Road Trail

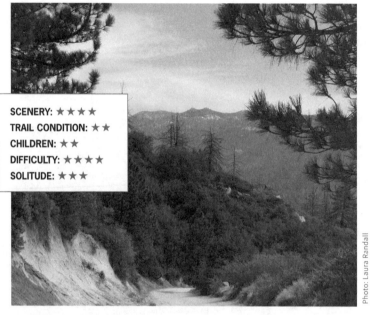

SCENERY: ★ ★ ★ ★
TRAIL CONDITION: ★ ★
CHILDREN: ★ ★
DIFFICULTY: ★ ★ ★ ★
SOLITUDE: ★ ★ ★

Photo: Laura Randall

HIKERS PICK UP ELEVATION GAIN—AND VIEWS—ALONG THE BLACK MOUNTAIN FIRE ROAD.

GPS TRAILHEAD COORDINATES: N33° 47.807' W116° 45.444'

DISTANCE & CONFIGURATION: 6-mile out-and-back

HIKING TIME: 5–6 hours

HIGHLIGHTS: Mountain views, manzanita, desert vegetation, fire lookout

ELEVATION GAIN: 2,400'

ACCESS: A wilderness permit is required on this trail; it's free and available at the Idyllwild Ranger Station, just down the road at 54270 Pine Crest Ave. There's a small free parking pullout and street parking near the trailhead.

MAPS: Available at Idyllwild Ranger Station

FACILITIES: None at trailhead

WHEELCHAIR ACCESS: None

COMMENTS: If you're hiking this trail in winter or early spring, watch out for iced-over sections of the trail. It makes for a dangerous combination with the trail's steepness.

CONTACTS: Idyllwild Ranger Station, 909-382-2921

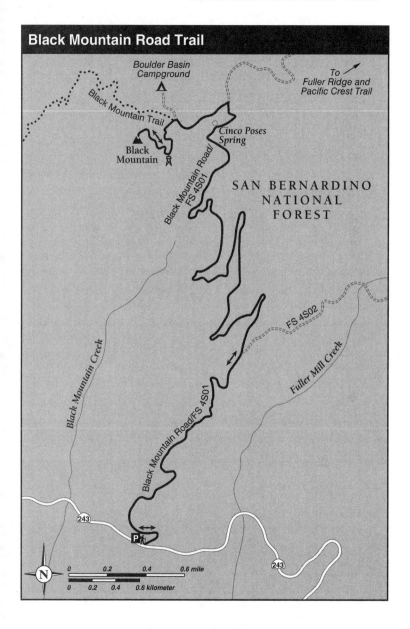

Black Mountain Road Trail

Boulder Basin
Campground

To
Fuller Ridge and
Pacific Crest Trail

Black Mountain Trail

Cinco Poses
Spring

Black
Mountain

Black Mountain Road/
FS 4S01

SAN BERNARDINO
NATIONAL
FOREST

Black Mountain Creek

FS 4S02

Fuller Mill Creek

Black Mountain Road/FS 4S01

243

0   0.2   0.4   0.6 mile

0   0.2   0.4   0.6 kilometer

N

P

243

Overview

This hike begins about 5 miles outside of Idyllwild Village and follows a wide fire road up a relentless 2,400 feet to a campground and lookout tower with panoramic views of the San Jacinto and San Bernardino mountains and San Gorgonio Pass. Some hikers prefer to do this hike in early spring, when the snow has melted but the road is still closed to vehicular traffic.

Route Details

Pick up the dirt fire road just beyond the US Forest Service sign for Black Mountain Road/Fuller Ridge Trail, on the north side of CA 243. The elevation gain kicks in immediately on this hike, which quickly envelopes you in a peaceful wilderness setting. It is almost entirely uphill until you reach Boulder Basin Campground. You will pass several unsigned trail splits; stay on the wide, winding fire road to reach Black Mountain Trail. The road is paved in some spots but is mostly packed dirt. Expect to see groves of oaks, pines, and scrub on the lower part of the trail. The pine forest gets denser and more beautiful the farther in you get. At about 4.1 miles, you will reach an unmarked clearing on the left. This is a staging area for the US Forest Service; no camping is allowed. Fringed by towering pines and large logs, it is a

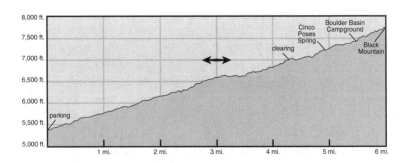

scenic place to stop and rest before continuing the remaining 2 miles to Black Mountain.

At about 5.3 miles, make a sharp left and follow the road about 0.25 mile past Boulder Basin Campground to its end. Take the paved path to the lookout tower, which is staffed by volunteers from May to September. If it's open, you are welcome to climb up the tower and enjoy the panoramic views and learn about fire prevention from the volunteers. On a clear day, you can see the Santa Rosa Mountains, San Jacinto Peak, San Gorgonio Pass, and even the Pacific Ocean. From here, you can retrace your route to the highway or set up camp at Boulder Basin and explore the other trails within the San Jacinto Mountains the next day.

Nearby Attractions

The road is open to four-wheel-drive vehicles in the late spring and summer, though you will need a National Forest Adventure Pass (see page 18) to leave your car anywhere within the forest boundaries. **Boulder Basin Campground (tinyurl.com/boulderbasin)** offers primitive single-family campsites in the shadow of the tower and makes a good base to explore other nearby trails, including Fuller Ridge and the Pacific Crest Trail. Reservations can be made at **recreation.gov,** but there are also some first-come, first-served sites available. The campground closes in winter and often doesn't reopen until mid-May.

Directions

From I-10, take Exit 100 for Idyllwild/CA 243 and follow CA 243 south up the mountain about 20 miles. About 2 miles past the Vista Grande Ranger Station, look for a sign for Black Mountain Road and turn left into the parking pullout. The road is usually closed to cars from November through April but is open for hiking year-round.

24 **Cactus Springs Trail**

SCENERY: ★ ★ ★
TRAIL CONDITION: ★ ★ ★
CHILDREN: ★
DIFFICULTY: ★ ★ ★
SOLITUDE: ★ ★ ★

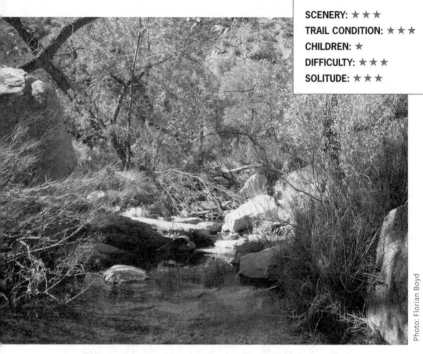

Photo: Florian Boyd

HORSETHIEF CREEK PROVIDES SHADE FOR HIKERS HEADING INTO THE
SANTA ROSA WILDERNESS AREA ON CACTUS SPRINGS TRAIL.

GPS TRAILHEAD COORDINATES: N33° 34.794' W116° 27.028'

DISTANCE & CONFIGURATION: 7-mile out-and-back

HIKING TIME: 4–6 hours

HIGHLIGHTS: Mountain views, manzanita, desert vegetation, seasonal stream

ELEVATION GAIN: 900'

ACCESS: A wilderness permit is required on this trail; it's free and available at the Idyllwild
Ranger Station (54270 Pine Crest Ave.) or in Palm Desert at the Santa Rosa and San
Jacinto National Monument Visitor Center (51500 CA 74).

MAPS: Available at Idyllwild Ranger Station

FACILITIES: None at trailhead

WHEELCHAIR ACCESS: None

COMMENTS: Dog owners and day hikers can take this trail to Horsethief Creek, rest a bit
in the shade, and then head back, which makes for a moderate 5-mile out-and-back hike.

CONTACTS: Idyllwild Ranger Station, 909-382-2921

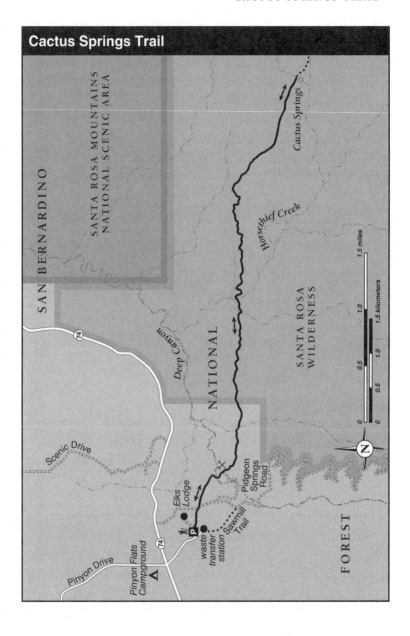

Cactus Springs Trail

SAN BERNARDINO

SANTA ROSA MOUNTAINS
NATIONAL SCENIC AREA

Cactus Springs

Horsethief Creek

Deep Canyon

NATIONAL

SANTA ROSA
WILDERNESS

Scenic Drive

Elks Lodge

Pidgeon Springs Road

Sawmill Trail

waste transfer station

Pinyon Flats Campground

Pinyon Drive

FOREST

0   0.5   1.0   1.5 miles
0   0.5   1.0   1.5 kilometers

Overview

This moderately challenging hike is the primary access route into the starkly beautiful Santa Rosa Wilderness. It zigzags through fields of sentinel yuccas and cacti, past an abandoned limestone quarry, and across a shaded creek, deep into the arid desert wilderness. The first 2.3 miles to Horsethief Creek are mostly downhill; then the trail heads out of the canyon for a rough and steep 4.5 miles to Cactus Springs (which is always dry) with views of the 6,500-foot pine-covered Martinez Mountain.

Route Details

Look for the trailhead sign at the east end of the parking lot and follow a wide dirt road east beyond the sign for Cactus Springs. An unsigned trail to the left leads to an Elks Lodge. Bikes aren't allowed here, but dogs and horses are. The first 2.5 miles are good for dogs, but after that the path gets rough and steep with many loose rocks. Continue on the dirt road about 0.2 mile to another sign for Cactus Springs. This marks the official start of the trail. If you continue straight on the dirt road, it will lead you a strenuous 9 miles up Sawmill Road to the base of Toro Peak.

For the 5-mile out-and-back, take the loose dirt trail to the left as it heads down into the canyon and past another trail sign and sign-in register. This is also where you should fill out a self-issued wilderness permit if you plan on camping overnight. The next 2 miles

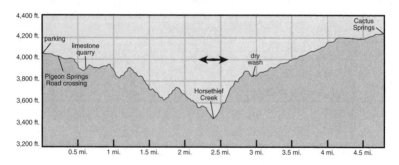

are an up-and-down trek (mostly down) past manzanita, desert sage, cacti, and other vegetation. There is little shade and only a few places to stop along this part of the trail. After about 0.5 mile, an old limestone quarry and its rusty machinery will come into view. The trail takes you farther down into the canyon, then up and around to the quarry, where you can examine the white and pink crystallized dolomite rocks that were mined here.

Continue east on the trail as it heads past the quarry and a small clearing to a sign that warns hikers to beware of HAZARDOUS CONDITIONS BEYOND THIS POINT. Most likely, the sign is referring to the loose gravel trail that can be quite slippery after a rainfall. Keep an eye out for rattlesnakes as you walk, especially during the hot weather months.

At 1.8 miles, Horsethief Creek comes into view below you to the left, and it's another 0.5 mile downhill to the creek. There are a few large rocks, fallen logs, and cottonwood trees at the crossing, marking the best place along the trail to rest and rehydrate or pitch a tent and spend the night. As the story goes, the creek got its name because 19th-century horse thieves used to hide the animals in this densely wooded area before driving them to the cities to sell.

From here the trail heads uphill for a steep quarter-mile to a mountain ridge, then follows a dry canyon wash for about 2 miles. The area really doesn't invite lingering, but stop for a moment to take in the solitude and desolate desert wilderness, and you'll begin to appreciate why the horse thieves liked to hide out here.

Keep in mind that the trip back will be tougher than the hike in—the elevation gain between Horsethief Creek and the trailhead is about 900 feet. Bring plenty of water and sunscreen. Though this is a popular and well-known trail, it doesn't get much traffic.

Nearby Attractions

Camp overnight at the year-round **Pinyon Flat Campground** ($8 a site, first-come, first-served) across the street from the trailhead. For updates on camping conditions in the area, contact the Santa Rosa and San Jacinto National Monument Visitor Center at 760-862-9984.

Directions

From CA 111 in Palm Desert, head south on CA 74 for about 14 miles to Pinyon Flat Campground. (From Idyllwild, it's about a 26-mile drive.) Turn left (south) at the sign for Sawmill Road, directly across from the Pinyon Flats Campground, follow it about 0.5 mile, and then make a left into the parking lot just before the waste transfer station. Park in the large lot and look for the sign for the Cactus Springs Trail at the lot's eastern edge.

Cedar Spring Trail

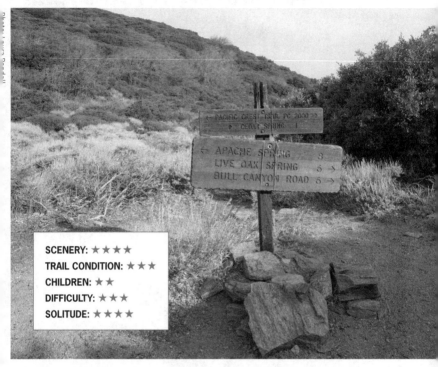

SCENERY: ★ ★ ★ ★
TRAIL CONDITION: ★ ★ ★
CHILDREN: ★ ★
DIFFICULTY: ★ ★ ★
SOLITUDE: ★ ★ ★ ★

THE CEDAR SPRING TRAIL TRAVERSES SWITCHBACKS AND QUIET PASTURES BEFORE CONNECTING TO THE PACIFIC CREST TRAIL AND OTHER PATHS.

GPS TRAILHEAD COORDINATES: N33° 39.246' W116° 35.378'

DISTANCE & CONFIGURATION: 4.4-mile out-and-back

HIKING TIME: 3 hours

HIGHLIGHTS: Mountain views, manzanita, views of Palm Springs and the Coachella Valley

ELEVATION GAIN: 1,400'

ACCESS: No wilderness permit is required on this trail. Dogs are allowed but should be kept on a leash for the first mile.

MAPS: Available at Idyllwild Ranger Station, 54270 Pine Crest Ave.

FACILITIES: None at trailhead

WHEELCHAIR ACCESS: None

COMMENTS: This road passes through parcels of private property for the first mile; be respectful of the NO TRESPASSING signs and stay on the trail.

CONTACTS: Idyllwild Ranger Station, 909-382-2921

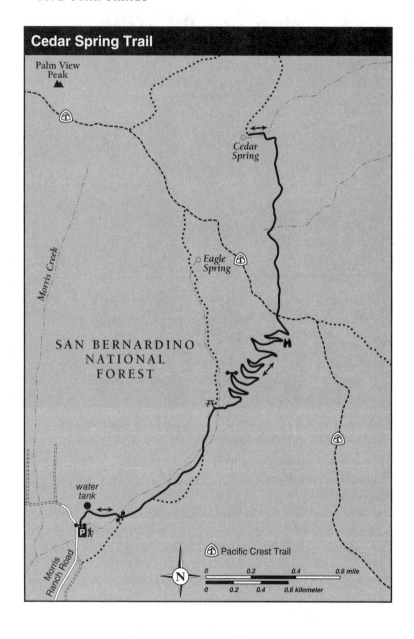

Cedar Spring Trail

Palm View Peak

Cedar Spring

Morris Creek

Eagle Spring

SAN BERNARDINO
NATIONAL
FOREST

water
tank

Morris Ranch Road

Pacific Crest Trail

N

| 0 | 0.2 | 0.4 | 0.6 mile |
| 0 | 0.2 | 0.4 | 0.6 kilometer |

Overview

This quiet out-and-back hike is one of my favorites in the Palm Springs area. It is easy to follow, provides a moderate cardio workout, and is marked by thick groves of manzanita and gorgeous views of both mountains and desert. It starts out traversing privately owned pastures, switchbacks up a mountain for 1.5 miles, and crosses the Pacific Crest Trail (PCT), which is closed to through-traffic at this point due to damages caused by wildfires in 2013. The hike can be done year-round, though the best times are spring and early fall.

Route Details

Walk through the unlocked gate on the right side of Morris Ranch Road and follow a dirt road northeast toward the mountains. At 0.25 mile, you will come to another unlocked gate; walk through it and continue following the dirt road up a gradual incline. The road starts to narrow and fill with loose rocks at this point, and it's well shaded by dense oaks and pines. Soon you'll come to a large sign indicating that Cedar Spring is 3 miles ahead. The road continues gently uphill past desert lavender, sage, manzanita, yucca, and paddle cactus.

At 0.8 mile, you'll pass two old picnic tables nestled in an attractive clearing. Continue walking as the road turns into a trail and veers east and heads through dense forest before ascending the mountainside

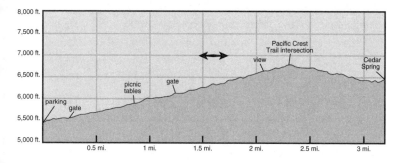

in long switchbacks. Just before you reach the 1-mile point, you'll come to a sign for the PCT (1.5 miles from here) and Cedar Spring (2.5 miles). The next 1.5 miles are a steady uphill climb accompanied by terrific views of Garner Valley and the San Jacinto Mountains. The trail skirts a seasonal stream before the switchbacks begin, though don't expect more than a trickle under drought conditions.

At 1.2 miles, you'll pass through the last of the unlocked gates; from here, the trail continues switchbacking up the mountain. At 2 miles, you'll pass a clearing with a few rocks and wide-open views of the mountains and the valley; this is one of the few places to stop and rest before the top of the mountain. The trail reaches a saddle at 2.2 miles and meets the PCT at a four-way junction. A natural wood bench is shaded by an oak tree tucked into one corner. At this point, elevation 6,800 feet, you've gained 1,400 feet from the trailhead.

Note: Due to a wildfire that swept through the area in 2013, the trail is closed at the PCT and points north, so the mile-long trail that leads to Cedar Spring Campground is indefinitely inaccessible, according to the Forest Service. Be prepared to turn around at this point and retrace your steps back to Morris Ranch Road.

Directions

From CA 111 in Palm Desert, follow CA 74 south about 19 miles to Morris Ranch Road. Make a right and follow the road about 3 miles to a sign for the Cedar Spring Trail on the left. Park on the side of the road, being mindful of the private driveways and NO TRESPASSING signs.

Alternate directions: The trail is about 10 miles from Idyllwild. Take CA 243 south from town about 4.5 miles until it meets CA 74 in Mountain Center. Turn left and follow CA 74 about 7 miles to Morris Ranch Road. Make a left and follow the road about 3 miles to a sign for the Cedar Spring Trail on the right. Park on the side of the road, being mindful of the private driveways and NO TRESPASSING signs. Call the San Jacinto Mountains Ranger Station at 909-659-2607 for more information about overnight-camping permits.

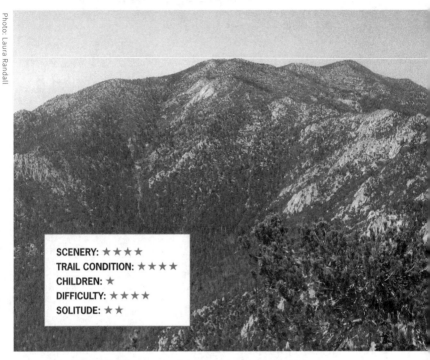

SCENERY: ★ ★ ★ ★
TRAIL CONDITION: ★ ★ ★ ★
CHILDREN: ★
DIFFICULTY: ★ ★ ★ ★
SOLITUDE: ★ ★

MOUNTAIN VIEWS REWARD HIKERS WHO MAKE IT TO THE TOP OF DEER SPRINGS TRAIL.

GPS TRAILHEAD COORDINATES: N33° 45.175' W116° 43.358'

DISTANCE & CONFIGURATION: 7.2-mile out-and-back

HIKING TIME: 3–4 hours

HIGHLIGHTS: Mountain views, manzanita, pine forest, rock formations

ELEVATION GAIN: 1,800'

ACCESS: A wilderness permit is required on this trail; it's free and available at the Idyllwild Ranger Station (54270 Pine Crest Ave.) or in Palm Desert at the Santa Rosa and San Jacinto National Monument Visitor Center (51500 CA 74).

MAPS: Available at Idyllwild Ranger Station

FACILITIES: Restrooms at the Idyllwild Nature Center, across the street from trailhead

WHEELCHAIR ACCESS: None

COMMENTS: Dogs aren't allowed beyond the first 0.25 mile of this trail.

CONTACTS: Idyllwild Ranger Station, 909-382-2921

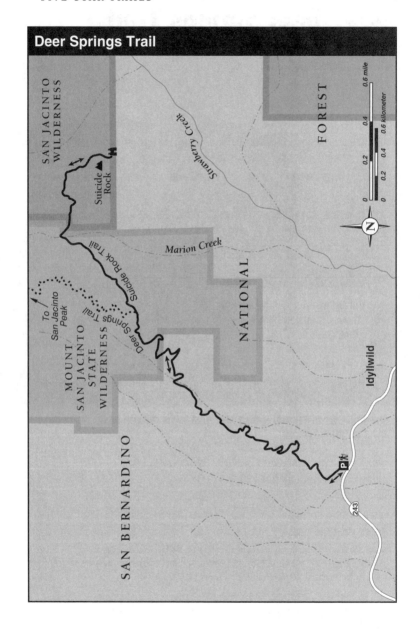

Deer Springs Trail

SAN JACINTO WILDERNESS

Suicide Rock

Strawberry Creek

Marion Creek

Suicide Rock Trail

To San Jacinto Peak

Deer Springs Trail

MOUNT SAN JACINTO STATE WILDERNESS

FOREST

NATIONAL

N

0   0.2   0.4   0.6 mile

0   0.2   0.4   0.6 kilometer

Idyllwild

P

243

SAN BERNARDINO

Overview

This strenuous hike heads up Deer Springs Trail via long switchbacks, then winds 1 mile east up to the top of Suicide Rock, a wide, open clearing with views of pine-covered mountains and Lily Rock. Easily accessible from downtown Idyllwild and CA 243, this is one of the area's most popular trails, according to the US Forest Service.

Route Details

Pick up any of the paths that lead out of the small dirt parking lot; they all funnel into the main Deer Springs Trail. Follow the narrow dirt trail as it heads north up a mountainside via long switchbacks. The first 0.25 mile is a little barren, but you'll start to see canyon live oaks, Coulter pines, and manzanita as you get deeper into the wilderness. At 0.25 mile, the Deer Springs Trail curves right and passes a sign warning that dogs aren't allowed beyond this point. At 0.8 mile, soon after you pass a sign for the San Jacinto State Park Wilderness, the trail splits. Go left to stay on Deer Springs Trail; the right path dead-ends at a small viewpoint.

The trail continues to switchback up the mountain for another 1.4 miles before reaching a junction and the turnoff for Suicide Rock. Turn right, then almost immediately left on a narrow, shaded trail up

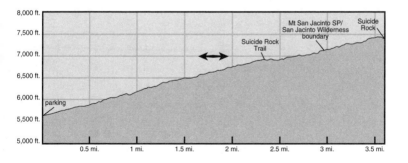

the mountain. Pass through the cut in a large fallen tree and continue another mile across Marion Creek to Suicide Rock. The elevation gain between the junction and Suicide Rock is about 500 feet. Expect to see plenty of purple San Jacinto lupine, manzanita, and buckwheat along this part of the trail.

The first half of the hike ends at the bleached cliffs of Suicide Rock. As the legend goes, the rock got its name after a Native American princess and her unsuitable lover threw themselves off the rock, à la Romeo and Juliet. A more believable piece of data: This is one of the top rock-climbing destinations in Southern California.

After resting and soaking up the panoramic views of Strawberry Valley, you have two options: (1) retrace your route to the parking lot or (2) retrace your route to the junction, then turn right and climb 2 more strenuous miles on the Deer Springs Trail to Strawberry Junction.

Directions

From downtown Idyllwild, drive north 1 mile on CA 243 to the sign for the Deer Springs Trail on the right. Turn right and park in the small dirt lot across the street from the Idyllwild Nature Center.

OPTION From I-10 in Banning, take Exit 100 for Idyllwild/CA 243 and head south up the mountain for about 25 miles. Look for the DEER SPRINGS TRAIL sign on the left side of the road. Turn left and park in the small dirt lot across the street from the Idyllwild Nature Center.

Devil's Slide Trail

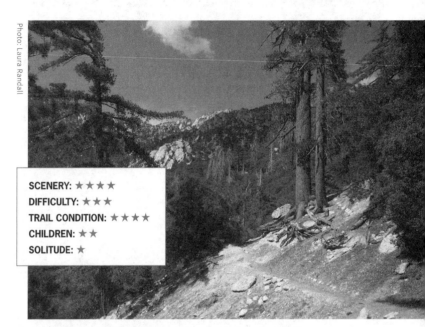

SCENERY: ★ ★ ★ ★
DIFFICULTY: ★ ★ ★
TRAIL CONDITION: ★ ★ ★ ★
CHILDREN: ★ ★
SOLITUDE: ★

**WELL-MAINTAINED SWITCHBACKS MAKE THE DEVIL'S SLIDE TRAIL
A FAVORITE MODERATE HIKE.**

GPS TRAILHEAD COORDINATES: N33° 45.859' W116° 41.142'

DISTANCE & CONFIGURATION: 5-mile out-and-back

HIKING TIME: 2–3 hours

HIGHLIGHTS: Scenic views of San Jacinto Mountains and Suicide Rock; pine forest; sheer rock walls

ELEVATION GAIN: 1,700'

ACCESS: A National Forest Adventure Pass is required to park here (see page 18). Hikers must also pick up a free wilderness permit at the Idyllwild Ranger Station, at 54270 Pine Crest Ave. in downtown Idyllwild.

MAPS: Available at Idyllwild Ranger Station

FACILITIES: Restrooms at Humber Park

WHEELCHAIR ACCESS: None

COMMENTS: You can also reach San Jacinto Peak from here by turning left at Saddle Junction and following the Saddle Junction Trail another 5.5 miles to the peak. This should only be attempted by experienced hikers prepared with maps and supplies.

CONTACTS: Idyllwild Ranger Station, 909-382-2921

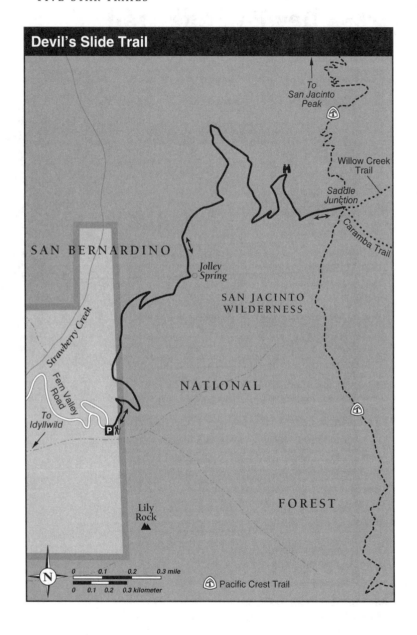

Devil's Slide Trail

To
San Jacinto
Peak

Willow Creek
Trail

Saddle
Junction

Caramba Trail

SAN BERNARDINO

Jolley
Spring

SAN JACINTO
WILDERNESS

Strawberry Creek

Fern Valley
Road

To
Idyllwild

NATIONAL

Lily
Rock

FOREST

N

0   0.1   0.2   0.3 mile
0   0.1   0.2   0.3 kilometer

Pacific Crest Trail

Overview

A series of moderately challenging switchbacks leads past scenic views of Lily Rock and pine-covered mountains to Saddle Junction, where you can pick up the Pacific Crest Trail or continue all the way to San Jacinto Peak. With a 1,700-foot elevation gain and an easy-to-follow trail, it's a good moderate hike that can be done in a couple of hours.

Route Details

Pick up the trailhead across from the restrooms in Humber Park. Look for the large sign marking the Devil's Slide Trail and follow the trail north into the boulder- and pine-covered wilderness. The trail gets its name from early-20th-century ranchers who took their cattle to the top to graze before a clear trail was blazed. You'll see why as you begin a steady ascent via long switchbacks on a singletrack trail of packed dirt and rocks. The busy parking area quickly fades from sight and is replaced by wide-open views and pine-covered mountains. The higher you get, the denser and rockier the surroundings get, with the dirt trail often giving way to natural rock steps as it continues up the mountain.

After about 1.5 miles of uphill hiking, the trail levels briefly and passes a small clearing on the right with a spectacular view of lush green mountains. This is one of the few places for hikers to stop

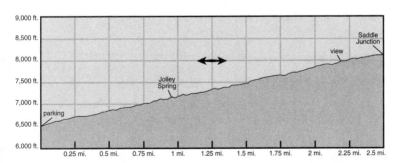

and rest along the trail. Continue another 0.5 mile to a huge boulder and another viewpoint with mountain vistas. I saw several hikers with dogs on this trail when I hiked it on a late Saturday afternoon. The dogs seemed to be having as much fun scrambling around the rocks and logs as the humans were.

From here the trail gets narrower and steeper as it switchbacks uphill another 0.25 mile to Saddle Junction. A sheer rock wall hugs one side of the path for a while just before you reach the saddle. At 2.5 miles, the trail opens to a wide and flat clearing shaded by towering sugar, Jeffrey, and ponderosa pines and strewn with logs and large rocks. This is a great place to stop and rest before heading back or going on to San Jacinto or Tahquitz Peak.

A sign marks the end of Devil's Slide Trail and its junction with several other San Jacinto Mountain trails. Camping is allowed 300 yards from the trail from this point on; most campers prefer to walk another mile to Skunk Cabbage Meadow or Willow Creek, where they can set up camp near a year-round stream. From Skunk Cabbage Meadow, it's about 4 miles to Long Valley and the Palm Springs Aerial Tramway. You can also turn left at the junction marking the end of the Devil's Slide Trail and follow the Pacific Crest Trail for about 3 miles, then turn right and continue another mile to campsites in Little Round Valleys. Be sure to pick up an overnight-camping permit at the Idyllwild Ranger Station and check with the staff about trail conditions. There is often snow on the ground as late as April or May up here.

Directions

From the Idyllwild Ranger Station (CA 243 at Pine Crest Avenue), head north and east 0.6 mile on Pine Crest Avenue to North Circle Drive. At the intersection, cross North Circle Drive (Pine Crest becomes South Circle Drive) and Strawberry Creek; then make an immediate left onto Fern Valley Road. Stay on Fern Valley Road for 1.9 miles (being careful not to veer off onto other residential roads) and follow the signs for Humber Park to the parking area.

Hurkey Creek Trail

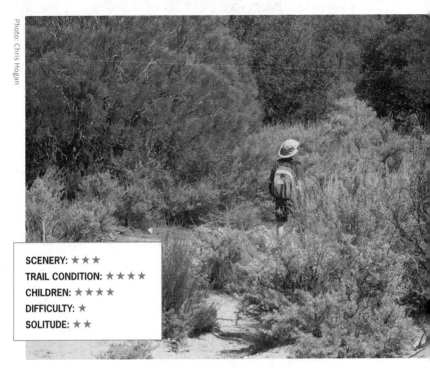

SCENERY: ★ ★ ★
TRAIL CONDITION: ★ ★ ★ ★
CHILDREN: ★ ★ ★ ★
DIFFICULTY: ★
SOLITUDE: ★ ★

DESERT VEGETATION SURROUNDS THE MOSTLY FLAT HURKEY CREEK TRAIL.

GPS TRAILHEAD COORDINATES: N33° 40.763' W116° 40.902'

DISTANCE & CONFIGURATION: 2-mile out-and-back

HIKING TIME: 45 minutes–1 hour

HIGHLIGHTS: Year-round stream, desert vegetation, mountain views

ELEVATION GAIN: 186'

ACCESS: Open to day hikers from sunrise to sunset. There is a small fee to park in the lot.

MAPS: Available at Idyllwild Ranger Station, 54270 Pine Crest Ave.

FACILITIES: Restrooms, water

WHEELCHAIR ACCESS: Yes

COMMENTS: Hurkey Creek is a stop on the **24 Hours of Adrenalin** endurance bike race, which takes place several times a year in spring and fall. Hikers will want to avoid this trail during those times. Check **24hoursofadrenalin.com** for exact dates.

CONTACTS: Idyllwild Ranger Station, 909-382-2921

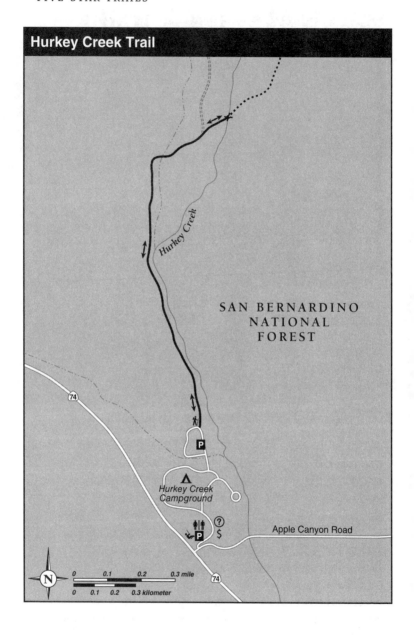

Hurkey Creek Trail

Hurkey Creek

SAN BERNARDINO
NATIONAL
FOREST

74

Hurkey Creek
Campground

Apple Canyon Road

74

| 0 | 0.1 | 0.2 | 0.3 mile |
| 0 | 0.1 | 0.2 | 0.3 kilometer |

N

Overview

This is a pleasant, easy walk past desert sage, lavender, manzanita, and a gurgling stream—perfect for children, dogs, and novice hikers. One of the best times to hike the trail is in spring, after a rainy winter, when wildflowers frame the views and the stream is robust with water. Be aware that the trail is also popular with mountain bikers, who pick it up on their way down the mountainside from Keen Ridge.

Route Details

Pick up the trailhead on the northern edge of the campground. Walk around the fire road gate and follow the trail north as it parallels Hurkey Creek. From here it's a flat 1-mile walk past desert vegetation—and wide-open views of the San Bernardino Mountains—to a small wooden bridge that crosses the creek. Most day hikers turn back here, although you can wander deeper into the San Bernardino Forest by continuing on the trail after crossing the bridge or take the trail to the left, just before you come to the bridge. Both trails head steeply uphill for several miles before looping back to CA 74; these trails are more popular with mountain bikers than with hikers.

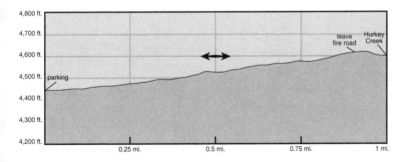

Directions

The trailhead is about an 8-mile drive from Idyllwild and 40 miles from Palm Springs. From Palm Springs, take CA 111 east to CA 74, then follow CA 74 south about 32 miles to Apple Canyon Road. Make a right, then bear left into Hurkey Creek Campground. Pay a small fee at the kiosk, where you can also pick up a map of the Hurkey Creek area, including the campground and trails, and park in the lot.

29 **Ramona Trail**

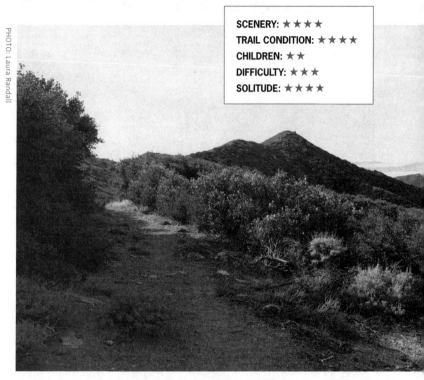

PHOTO: Laura Randall

SCENERY: ★ ★ ★ ★
TRAIL CONDITION: ★ ★ ★ ★
CHILDREN: ★ ★
DIFFICULTY: ★ ★ ★
SOLITUDE: ★ ★ ★ ★

THE RAMONA TRAIL OFFERS A GRADUAL TRANSITION FROM DESERT LANDSCAPE TO PINE FORESTS.

GPS TRAILHEAD COORDINATES: N33° 37.273' W116° 38.033'

DISTANCE & CONFIGURATION: 8-mile out-and-back

HIKING TIME: 3–4 hours

HIGHLIGHTS: Mountain views, manzanita, ribbonwood, pine forest, desert vegetation

ELEVATION GAIN: 1,700'

ACCESS: No wilderness permit is required for day hikers on this trail, though a National Forest Adventure Pass (see page 18) is required to park in the lot.

MAPS: Available at Idyllwild Ranger Station, 54270 Pine Crest Ave.

FACILITIES: Restrooms, water

WHEELCHAIR ACCESS: Yes

COMMENTS: Dogs are allowed on this trail.

CONTACTS: Idyllwild Ranger Station, 909-382-2921

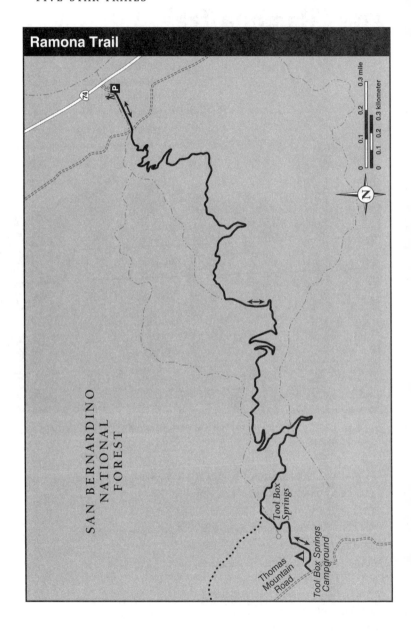

Overview

This well-maintained trail near Lake Hemet is enhanced by beautiful views of the San Jacinto Mountains and a gradual transition from desert landscape to dense pine forest. It begins just off CA 74 and follows several miles of switchbacks up a mountainside covered in pine, manzanita, ribbonwood, and huge rocks to a series of pristine campsites. Day hikers can follow the trail 4 miles to Tool Box Springs Campground, then retrace their route to the trailhead for a moderate out-and-back hike with views that are just as breathtaking on the way back down as when going up. Start early in the morning if you can, especially in summer, and bring plenty of water and sunscreen any time of the year.

Route Details

Access the Ramona Trail by following the dirt road past a gate on the northwest corner of the parking lot. After 50 yards or so, look for a narrow trail that branches left and follow that another 50 yards to a sign for the Ramona Trail. The singletrack trail immediately begins switchbacking uphill past manzanita, ribbonwood, and small clusters of cacti. You'll gain elevation at a steady pace from here on, for a total of 1,700 feet to Tool Box Springs; expect little or no shade on the first mile. The mountain views that make this trail one of my favorites soon appear

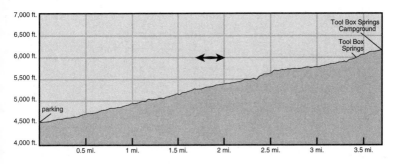

and stay with you for much of the way to the top. At about 0.6 mile, the trail skirts a small clearing—this is one of the few places to stop and rest along the way. As you approach 1 mile, the sandy trail gives way to larger rocks and gravel and starts to leave the desert landscape behind. After another mile or so of switchbacking, the trail gets shadier, the pine trees that flank it are noticeably bigger and denser, and oak trees dot the landscape. The rocks are also larger and more striking the farther in you go. You may encounter a couple of fallen logs blocking the path—they are fairly easy for hikers to climb over but more of a hassle for the cyclists and equestrians who also use the trail.

As you near Tool Box Springs, the trail levels for longer stretches and wanders through dense forest before splitting into two separate trails at 3.6 miles. Just before a sign for the Ramona Trail, there is a narrow trail on the right marked by a small post. Take that unnamed trail uphill for about 2 miles to a wide clearing with a few primitive campsites and picnic tables; this trail eventually leads to Thomas Mountain.

Day hikers can retrace their route to the Ramona Trail parking lot.

Directions

From CA 111 in Palm Desert, follow CA 74 south about 21 miles, past Pinyon Flats Campground and Morris Ranch Road. Look for a sign for the Ramona Trail to Tool Box Springs, and turn left into a small dirt parking lot. A National Forest Adventure Pass (see page 18) is required to park.

From downtown Idyllwild, take CA 243 south about 4.5 miles until it meets CA 74 in Mountain Center. Turn left and follow CA 74 about 5 miles to the sign for the Ramona Trail.

30

San Jacinto Peak

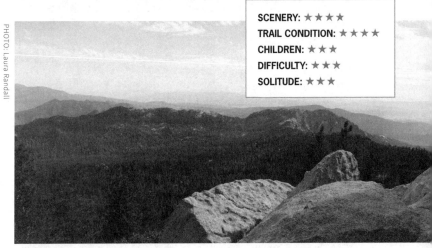

SCENERY: ★ ★ ★ ★
TRAIL CONDITION: ★ ★ ★ ★
CHILDREN: ★ ★
DIFFICULTY: ★ ★ ★
SOLITUDE: ★ ★ ★

PHOTO: Laura Randall

HIKERS TAKE IN VIEWS OF THE SANTA ROSA MOUNTAINS ALONG THE TRAIL TO SAN JACINTO PEAK.

GPS TRAIL COORDINATES: N33° 48.900' W116° 38.350'

DISTANCE & CONFIGURATION: 11-mile out-and-back

HIKING TIME: 6–7 hours

HIGHLIGHTS: Panoramic mountain and desert views, pine forest, grassy meadows, ancient rocks

ELEVATION GAIN: 2,300'

ACCESS: This hike requires a ride on the Palm Springs Aerial Tramway ($24.95 per adult, $16.95 per child ages 3–12; see Directions for operating hours). The tram whisks you 8,500 feet from the desert floor to Mount San Jacinto State Park, with a corresponding temperature drop of as much as 30 degrees. If you want to day-hike, arrive early and pick up a free wilderness permit at the Long Valley Ranger Station. For information on how to pick up an advance permit, visit **pstramway.com/wilderness-permits.html.**

MAPS: Available at Tramway Station and Palm Springs Bureau of Tourism

FACILITIES: Restrooms, water

WHEELCHAIR ACCESS: Limited to areas around Tramway Station

COMMENTS: If you hike in the winter or spring, bring waterproof boots and other raingear. Trail sections that hug rain-swollen creeks are often wet and slippery. Layered clothing is a good idea year-round.

CONTACTS: Palm Springs Tramway, 760-325-1391 or **pstramway.com;** Palm Springs Bureau of Tourism, 760-778-8415, **visitpalmsprings.com.** For hiking information, write Mount San Jacinto State Park, PO Box 308, 25905 CA 243, Idyllwild, CA 92549; call 951-659-2607 or visit **tinyurl.com/mtsanjacintosp.**

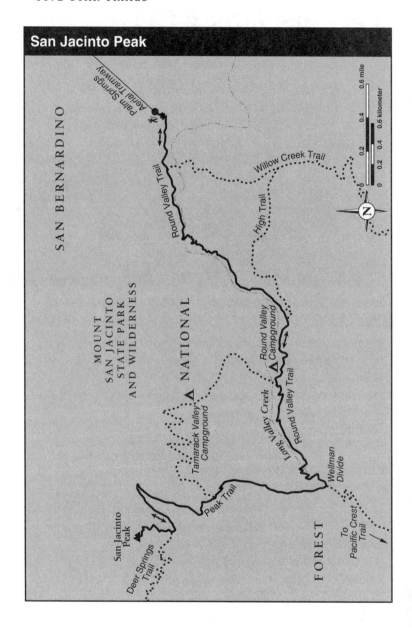

San Jacinto Peak

SAN BERNARDINO

Palm Springs Aerial Tramway

Round Valley Trail

Willow Creek Trail

High Trail

MOUNT SAN JACINTO STATE PARK AND WILDERNESS

NATIONAL

Round Valley Campground

Tamarack Valley Campground

Low Valley Creek

Round Valley Trail

Wellman Divide

Peak Trail

San Jacinto Peak

Deer Springs Trail

FOREST

To Pacific Crest Trail

N

0   0.2   0.4   0.6 mile
0   0.2   0.4   0.6 kilometer

Overview

The first 2.5 miles of this out-and-back hike are a gradual climb through pine forest and grassy meadows to Round Valley Campground. At Wellman Divide, the trail leads to stunning views of the Santa Rosa Mountains, then gives way to even better vistas of mountains, desert, and ancient rocks—views that stay with you for the remainder of the climb. The total elevation gain of 2,300 feet is gradual but unrelenting.

Route Details

At 10,834 feet, San Jacinto Peak is the second-highest peak in Southern California. Before heading out, stop at the park office on the ground level of the tramway station for a free map. Head outside and follow the concrete sidewalk as it descends to the valley below. At 1.1 miles, you'll come to a sign for Round Valley and San Jacinto Peak. Follow the trail to the left as it skirts a massive fallen tree trunk. From here it's another mile through dense woodland and between cragged rocks to Round Valley Campground, a flat clearing with 28 sites, pit toilets, and water (though it must be purified before drinking). Set up camp here or continue another half-mile uphill to Tamarack Valley Campground, where there are 12 campsites. Expect to see

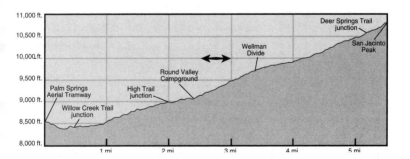

mule deer, coyotes, black-tailed jackrabbits, and dozens of species of birds in this area. Expect few hikers beyond this point.

Tired day hikers may be tempted to stop and have lunch at Round Valley, but it's worth it to continue on the main trail another mile to Wellman Divide, where (at 9,700 feet), there are exquisite views and large rocks that invite sitting. From here look east for a view of Tahquitz Peak, the Santa Rosa mountain range, and even the Salton Sea. This is also a starting point for the Saddle Junction Trail.

Leaving Wellman Divide, the trail dips north into a rock-strewn pine forest for about a mile, then leaves the forest and follows a manzanita-covered mountain ridge almost the rest of the way to San Jacinto Peak.

After nearly 3 steadily uphill miles, the trail turns sharply to the left and ends just below the peak's summit. Here you'll find a small stone shelter, built by the California Conservation Corps in 1935, which contains bunk beds, a stove, and (usually) the trail register. Anyone can use the cabin.

From the stone cabin, it's a 100-yard climb up a pile of boulders (keep to the left when in doubt) to the peak. A small, brown sign atop the highest rock marks the summit. From here you'll have views of Mount San Gorgonio, the San Bernardino Mountains, the entire Coachella Valley, and even the Pacific Ocean and Inland Empire on a clear day. The naturalist John Muir called it "the most sublime spectacle to be found anywhere on this earth."

The rocky and windy conditions at the summit make camping here difficult, though some hardy souls have attempted it. There are tales of people hiking down the peak at 3 a.m. to take shelter in the stone hut because they couldn't tolerate the cold and strong winds. No matter where you choose to camp, though, the view from the summit is likely one of the best you'll ever experience.

The return trip to Round Valley Campground is an easy downhill trek of 3.5 miles, and then it's another 2.5 miles back to the tramway station. Just make sure you allow for plenty of time to get there before dark.

Directions

From I-10 in Palm Springs, take Exit 120 and drive south on Indian Canyon Drive about 3.5 miles. At West San Rafael Road, turn right (west) and drive 0.7 mile. Keep straight on San Rafael across Palm Canyon Drive (CA 111). San Rafael becomes Tramway Road after the intersection; follow Tramway about 4 miles to the Palm Springs Aerial Tramway's Valley Station, and park in the lot. Starting at 10 a.m. Monday–Friday and at 8 a.m. on weekends and holidays, tramway cars depart at least every half-hour. The last tram car departs at 9:45 p.m. The tramway is typically closed for maintenance for several days in September. For more information, call 760-325-1391 or visit **pstramway.com.**

31

South Ridge Trail

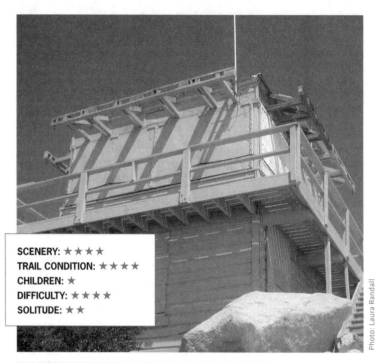

SCENERY: ★ ★ ★ ★
TRAIL CONDITION: ★ ★ ★ ★
CHILDREN: ★
DIFFICULTY: ★ ★ ★ ★
SOLITUDE: ★ ★

Photo: Laura Randall

**THE STRENUOUS SOUTH RIDGE TRAIL ENDS AT THE BASE OF A
FIRE LOOKOUT TOWER.**

GPS TRAILHEAD COORDINATES: N33° 44.094' W116° 41.768'

DISTANCE & CONFIGURATION: 7.2-mile out-and-back

HIKING TIME: 4–5 hours

HIGHLIGHTS: Tahquitz Peak, historic fire lookout, views of Palm Springs and the
Coachella Valley, dramatic rock formations

ELEVATION GAIN: 2,300'

ACCESS: Hikers must obtain a free wilderness permit for this trail, available near the
trailhead at the Idyllwild Ranger Station, at 54270 Pine Crest Ave. in downtown Idyllwild.

MAPS: Available at Idyllwild Ranger Station

FACILITIES: Restrooms, water

WHEELCHAIR ACCESS: None

COMMENTS: This trail is best hiked on a clear spring or fall day; the views it is known for
can be greatly obscured on hazy days.

CONTACTS: Idyllwild Ranger Station, 909-382-2921

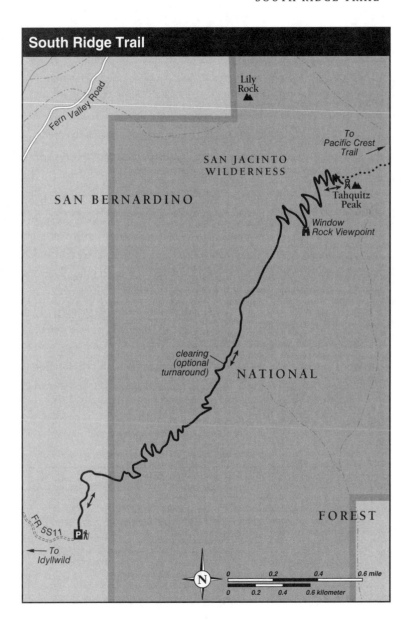

South Ridge Trail

Lily Rock

Fern Valley Road

To Pacific Crest Trail →

SAN JACINTO WILDERNESS

SAN BERNARDINO

Tahquitz Peak

Window Rock Viewpoint

clearing (optional turnaround)

NATIONAL

FOREST

FR 5S11

P

← To Idyllwild

N

| 0 | 0.2 | 0.4 | 0.6 mile |

| 0 | 0.2 | 0.4 | 0.6 kilometer |

Overview

This strenuous hike near the center of Idyllwild leads to Tahquitz Peak, the second-highest peak in California, and a lookout tower with sweeping views of the Palm Springs area, the San Jacinto Mountains, and even the Channel Islands. The total elevation gain is 2,300 feet. This is a favorite trail of several US Forest Service rangers because the scenic views begin almost immediately. You can make this hike as short or as long as you want and still be rewarded with memorable views.

Route Details

Look for the sign for the South Ridge Trail at the north corner of the parking area. Follow the trail into a dense forest of pine, spruce, and manzanita. Soon you'll pass a large wooden sign welcoming you to the San Jacinto Wilderness. The next mile follows a series of moderate switchbacks uphill past live oaks, manzanita, and many rocky outcroppings. After approximately 1.5 miles, the trail levels for about a mile and passes through a wide rocky clearing before resuming a strenuous uphill course, via switchbacks, to the peak. Just before the switchbacks begin, you'll come to a wide clearing with great views of the mountains to the west. This is a good turnaround point for those looking for a shorter, moderate hike. At 2.6 miles, you'll come to

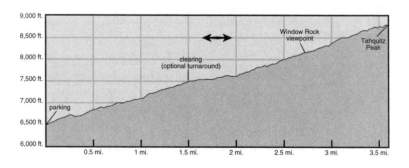

Window Rock, a striking viewpoint framed by several large boulders. One ranger likes to do this as a sunrise hike, arriving at the trailhead before dawn and hiking up to Window Rock in time to watch the sun come up over the Garner Valley. "You'll never seen another sunrise like it again," he told me.

The next mile is a strenuous climb via switchbacks to Tahquitz Peak. At 3.6 miles, you'll reach a three-way junction—follow the trail to the right to get to Tahquitz Peak; the trail to Saddle Junction, which goes straight, leads to the Pacific Crest Trail and Tahquitz Valley. From the junction, it's a short uphill walk to the base of a fire lookout tower, where you can rest and refuel before heading back. The views from the tower's base are superb, but you can climb the steps to the deck of the lookout for an even better vantage point. The lookout is closed during the winter and early spring but is staffed by volunteers from May to September.

Beware of rattlesnakes on the trail; they're a common sight during the hot summer and fall months. This is a year-round trail, but keep in mind that it can get quite hot in summer and be covered with ice and snow during winter. Check with the Idyllwild Ranger Station for updates and road conditions.

Directions

From downtown Idyllwild, drive south 0.7 mile on CA 243 to Saunders Meadow Road (the Mile High Cafe is on the corner). Turn left and follow the road 0.9 mile uphill to Pine Avenue. Make a left on Pine, then a right on Tahquitz View Drive. Follow the paved road until it ends at a sign for the South Ridge Trail. Turn right and take unpaved Forest Road 5S11 up a steep mile to the trailhead. If you don't have a four-wheel-drive vehicle, park on the street just below the fire road's entrance, being mindful of private property and NO TRESPASSING signs. This will add another strenuous uphill mile to the hike.

Appendix A: Outdoor Retailers

BIG 5 SPORTING GOODS
big5sportinggoods.com
2465 E. Palm Canyon Dr.
Palm Springs, CA
760-325-0255

31033 Date Palm Dr.
Cathedral City, CA
760-202-6702

DICK'S SPORTING GOODS
72-840 CA 111
Palm Desert, CA 92260
760-340-3526

ROUGH RIDERS SPORTING GOODS
roughriderssportinggoods.com
54245 N. Circle Dr.
Idyllwild, CA 92549
951-659-4043

72-840 CA 111
Palm Desert, CA 92260
760-340-3526

SPORTS AUTHORITY
sportsauthority.com
72-519 CA 111
Palm Desert, CA 92260
760-773-3270

Appendix B:
Map Resources

DESERT MAP AND AERIAL PHOTO
desertmapandaerial.com
73-612 CA 111
Palm Desert, CA 92260
760-346-1101

Carries a huge selection of books, topographic maps, and other resource materials. Desert Map and Aerial also sells the National Forest Adventure Pass (see page 17) in day and annual forms.

US GEOLOGICAL SURVEY
nationalmap.gov, usgs.gov

Appendix C:
Hiking Clubs

Local hiking groups meet online as well as on the trail. Nonmembers are welcome.

COACHELLA VALLEY HIKING CLUB
cvhikingclub.net
PO Box 10750
Palm Desert, CA 92255

DESERT TRAILS HIKING CLUB
deserttrailshiking.com
PO Box 10401
Palm Desert, CA 92255

THE MT. SAN JACINTO HIKING MEETUP GROUP
meetup.com/hiking-coachella-valley

Index

Page references followed by *m* indicate a map.

About the Author

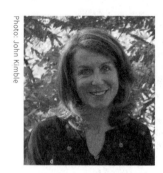

A native of suburban Philadelphia, **LAURA RANDALL** lived in Washington, D.C., and San Juan, Puerto Rico, before moving to Southern California in 1999. Her byline can be found in a variety of newspapers, consumer magazines, and websites, including the *Los Angeles Times*, the *Washington Post,* and *Sunset.* Her other books for Menasha Ridge Press are *60 Hikes Within 60 Miles: Los Angeles* and *Peaceful Places: Los Angeles.* She lives in Los Angeles.